The Millionaire Code:

Unlocking Your Financial Personality and Making More Money

per Buffingt

By

Perry W. Buffington, Ph.D.
Willa S. Presmanes, M.Ed., M.A.

*Willa Plesman
Keep in touch
through themillionairecode
.com*

A Southern Mountains Press Book

The Millionaire Code:
Unlocking Your Financial Personality
and Making More Money

A Southern Mountains Press Book/January 2003
All Rights Reserved
Copyright © 2003
Perry W. Buffington, Ph.D. & Willa S. Presmanes, M.Ed., M.A.

ISBN: 0-9723963-1-4

The information in this book is not a substitute for medical, psychological, legal, financial, or other professional advice or services. This book is for entertainment purposes only. Although it may
be helpful, it is sold for information purposes only.

The authors have made every effort to ensure that the information
in the book is accurate and complete. Neither the authors nor the
publisher will be held accountable for the use or misuse of the
information contained in this book.

Acknowledgements

We wish to thank family, friends and clients who examined and shared their personal **Millionaire Codes** so that we might share the wealth and teach others. We especially thank featured autobiographers who bravely recorded their specific weaknesses as well as their strengths in their success journeys. Knowing personality flaws and detailing how to lean toward strengths validates their work for those of us with similar dreams, interests and strengths. We also thank our editor and publisher Larry Chilnick who pushed and pulled us to truly personalize the **Millionaire Codes** for you, our readers.

Table of Contents

Introduction: Never Think About Money The Same Way!

Could you use a little extra cash?

Do you need more money?

It's not a trick question. The answer is "Who doesn't!" Money makes the world go round; and without it, life can come to an almost dead stop. And it's absolutely true. Money can't buy happiness, but it sure does make life's depression easier to swallow.

But here's the real query: Do you know where to find more money? Sure, you could work longer hours, take an extra job, inherit a fortune, win the lottery, marry money, win political office, invent the next fad, and/or rob a bank. You could take both fame and fortune by the napes of their neck and "Shake a living out of them." Fortunately, there's an easier way, certainly a more legal way, and maybe even a God-given way. To find more money, start close at hand.

So, where is this "magic" rich-in-cash place?

Would you be surprised if we told you your "secret money place" is tucked away in the neither-so-deep-nor-dark recesses of your personality? Would you be surprised if we told you your genetic brain wiring may just unravel the code, unlock the secrets of amassing wealth, working smarter, enjoying life more, getting along better with the love of your life, as well as living a healthier life?

Sounds too good to be true? Well, this is one time when it's not only too good, but too true, too! Never the less, it takes work, but not as much as you think! It takes a commitment, but not as much as you expect. It will require you to remove your blinders and understand how your old behaviors may be costing you big bucks. It will teach you a new way to think and behave, one that is more compatible with who you really are as opposed to who you think others think you are. No double talk and certainly no get-rich-quick scheme, this is simply a twist on the philosophic maxim: "Know yourself."

In this case, we're going to introduce you to and encourage you to "Know your '**Millionaire Code**.'" It's the first step in understanding your financial personality. It's possible. Others have unraveled this mystery, achieved financial freedom, even peace of mind, and you can, too. It's called "**The Millionaire Code**." Simply put, it's a way to unlock your financial personality and make more money. By identifying your **Millionaire Code**, you'll understand what we call your "financial DNA" —**D**ollars, **N**umbers and **A**ttitude. We'll help you hold a mirror up to both your banking accounts and yourself. Soon, you'll understand how you see money, how you pull it to you, how you push it away, how you attract it, how you spend it (or over-spend it), how you save it, even how you use it to buy peace, pleasure, problem solutions, or bully others. Once you see through the looking glass, you'll be in control of your money, rather than your money controlling you!

Here's how it all works. First, you'll be asked to answer sixteen short, even fun questions. Next, your score will place you in one of four money personality groups or **Millionaire Codes**:

- The Peacemaker
- The Pleasure Seeker
- The Problem Solver
- The Powerbroker

Once you know your "code," the rest of this book provides very specific information, very clear steps to help both you and your partner better handle cash. When you finish this book, you'll see money differently, approach it with more respect, and trust your instincts with it more than ever before.

By now, you're probably wondering: "Where did we get all this?" Well, "**The Millionaire Code**" started with a mild-mannered question from an audience member.

Following a lecture about four years ago, one of the country's top-100 certified financial planners asked us to apply our experience with creativity and personality strengths/weaknesses to financial personality profiling. Some of his clients had him stumped! He was very successful investing large sums of money for his clients, but someone in the family group always wanted more or something different — no one ever saw money the same way and was even mad they did not get it. He didn't know what to think, and while we had no immediate answers, he certainly got us looking back over our work and thinking out loud.

On the day of his question, here's what we knew. Our experience, working with people who have varied goals as well as multiple problems in their lives, had revealed three things. (1) Money is an issue in everyone's life in one way or another, regardless of how much or how little they earn. After all, it rains in everybody's life sometime. In addition, no two people in a close relationship think about money the same way. (2) Money is a vehicle to help us get where we want to go and needs to be discussed up front, but the subject of money is still a taboo subject in many relationships. To better understand the "taboo," we listened to young singles, couples, divorced men and women, single parents and virtually every other permutation of a "family" today. Then we researched the results of large-scale studies and concluded a third truth: (3) There seems to be a clear pattern of thinking and behavior where money, wants and needs are concerned that matched the personality characteristics of our clients. Armed with that new piece of information, and over a four-year period of time, we collected information that shed light on how personality and money worked symbiotically.

We found that (1) the personality types or **Millionaire Codes** listed above had both strengths and weaknesses that conflicted and prevented them from attaining as much success as they could muster. One was canceling out the other. (2) Our literature review also discovered that the biographies of wealthy and successful people revealed that many of them cycled between strengths and weaknesses for years before overcoming their negative personality weaknesses. Only when they used their financial personality strengths to rebound from loss did they amass fortunes and fame.

Finally, (3) all of these successful people had nothing in common regarding race, gender or ethnic background. But they did use their personality strengths to succeed. There was, we thought, and to borrow from the biological times, a whole new DNA code — Dollars, Numbers & Attitude that these "dollar scholars" possessed.

But if they had it—did everyone?

After we had enough data, we developed **The Millionaire Code** Questionnaire and a self-scoring form found in chapter three in this book. After we administered this test to our clients, the four patterns emerged. Once we knew how their personality saw money, then it was easy to help them better handle money. Many of their success stories are presented throughout the pages of this book. Also, this is a book for both you and your partner. Our research has confirmed that frequently money-DNA opposites attract. We show you how to make this work; and also, what happens when "birds of a feather flock together," those with similar money-DNA, join into partnerships.

Finally, because your health status affects your money directly and indirectly, we have looked at the impact of money-DNA on your health; and in Chapter 12, we tell you how to reduce stress so you can be financially healthy, wealthy and wise. After all, we regularly try to increase our resistance to illness and reduce our genetically programmed health risks, why not do the same things with money?

Everyone we have counseled wants to change or at least take charge of their financial situation and achieve financial security if not millionaire status. We know, just like the physician who looks at your family history, that this book can predict your current chance of success and give you a new start on the road to financial health. You have to do the rest — and we know you can!

Perry W. Buffington, Ph.D.

Willa S. Presmanes, M.Ed., M.A.

CHAPTER ONE

The Millionaire Code

1

Why did you buy that new car when your present car had only 50,000 miles on it? Why did you buy that "can't miss" stock in a rollercoaster atmosphere of corporate uncertainty at best? Why did you refinance your home after you saw some talking head on TV suggest that "now was the best time in history" to do so?

Sound familiar? Are you kicking yourself for one thing or another, ... "a big financial mistake?" Regrets? We all have them. Are you baffled because you seem to be absent from the right place at the right time, to make money, but you *are* right there to lose it?

The answers to these questions, and many others revealed in this book, are found by "unlocking your financial personality." No one wants to sabotage finances. However, that is exactly what so many of us do. Our thoughts and behavior with money have the power to either reel in debt or abundance. The result has everything to do with our "financial personality DNA" (**D**ollars, **N**umbers and **A**ttitude), your current behavior with money or what we dub **The Millionaire Code**.

This book tells you how to unlock your personal Code, how that step can help you make more money along with solid, rational choices — ones you won't regret when faced with personal financial decisions like those above. By answering 16 direct questions (developed by the authors in Chapter Three) you can tap into your strengths and weaknesses when it comes to money management and make positive, wealth enhancing changes. Despite each day's headlines unexpectedly revealing another stomach churning economic report, you still can pursue and capture financial security.

Your **Millionaire Code** identifies you as a blend of what we call a **Peacemaker, Powerbroker, Problem Solver,** or **Pleasure Seeker.** This code unlocks practical, useful information that will improve your financial status. You will also learn why you aren't — yet — a member of a small group of people (3.5% of the population called "The 3.5 Club") whose net worth is $1,000,000 in assets, excluding their place of residence, less liabilities such as the mortgage, secured and unsecured loans.

Is Life Only About Money?

Let's be honest with each other.

Do you want to be in the right place at the right time next time? Do you want to be a millionaire or at least very secure financially? Who doesn't? Be honest. Isn't the problem that you do want to obtain and retain as much wealth as possible, but you actually don't know how to do it. Maybe you even bought a lottery ticket (or two)?

The facts are that lottery sales and the number of vendors, including charitable lotteries, have doubled in the last decade. The typical lotto player spends about $800 a year for their chance to win it big without working for it. A lot of players spend much more and some play routinely smaller amounts. They just don't understand the reality of it. Factually, they have a far greater, better chance of being killed in a car crash on their way to buy the ticket than they do actually winning the big game.

Research shows that this is the way with most people. They're looking for something outside of themselves to bring them wealth. It never dawns on them that the answer to their money questions is located in their own brain, and they can see it in their behavior — if they'll just look.

So, why don't they look inside their own head for answers? Frankly, it's typically not the first place most people look to solve *any* problem. Perhaps they don't trust their own abilities, or maybe they don't think they have what it takes. Then there are those who believe that luck is a more powerful force in their life than their own skills. Others just reconcile themselves to the fact that they're just not capable of achieving money the old fashioned way —

earning and saving it. Instead, they settle for following the herd's tail lights in to town in the early morning and out again every evening, earning their living times forty hours a week (plus), and wondering why they can't get ahead. As a result, they can't indulge themselves and wish for million dollar fantasies. In reality, they'd settle for less. Researchers have found that the average in-debt John or Jane Doe believes that $50,000 would solve all of their financial problems. In today's economy, that's not a huge figure, but in many people's way of thinking $50,000 might as well be $50,000,000.

What to do to achieve a positive financial end? As we said, many look to the lottery, pretty much wasted money. There's always a new tax deferred savings plan that may be a smart idea, but relatively few can qualify for. Others actually hang around waiting for an inheritance, but that hardly satisfies here-and-now burning issues. Few know the secret of how to unlock the financial personality — or *their very own code of millionaire behavior*. The ones who learn that through this book are the ones who will get ahead and stay ahead, maybe even find themselves initiated into "The 3.5 Club."

The best place to start unlocking your inherent abilities is to evaluate your own mental approach to dollars and numbers, along with your attitude toward finances (your D, N, and A). Fortunately there's a way to do just that. Start by looking at your everyday, typical behavior because your behavior with money is showing. That's what this book is all about. Think of it as a guidebook, one that will help you discover and understand your own Money DNA. When you do, you'll begin to see a method to any money madness. It's all in your **Millionaire Code**, and it's not hiding, you've just misplaced it.

The More You Know the More You Keep

Knowing and understanding your **Millionaire Code** brings you more than just financial security. Understanding how your personality affects your financial decisions ultimately reduces stress when you have to make a decision. For example, financial decisions are rarely made in a vacuum. Frequently important decisions involve large purchases such as homes and automobiles where a spouse or another person is involved. It is almost guaranteed that their **Millionaire Code** is not the same as yours. In fact, data shows that financial disputes are among the most divisive within families.

Using the information will change that dynamic. Because you recognize your disparate **Millionaire Codes** and your strengths and weaknesses in one or more of the categories, you will learn how to work together to solve financial challenges.

Is This Really As Simple As It Seems?

The Millionaire Code is based on numerous studies and original research carried out by the authors as advisors to diverse groups such as "nearly-wed" couples, high-income executives, stockbrokers, and government officials charged with handling public funds. These studies and work with groups and individuals have also revealed a great deal about the public's somewhat ambiguous approach to the subject of "money" even though scientists have embraced many other facets of personality or genetic based research as solutions to a variety of problems.

Why is this?

As the 21st century dawns few will argue that one of the great scientific breakthroughs that will affect our lives in many, many ways are methods of unlocking the secrets our genetic codes hold. Researchers hope to predict markers that will indicate risk of serious disease and with that information create cures that prevent diabetes, cancer, heart disorders, birth defects and many other problems. Despite some controversy, it is not likely that these research pathways will stop and, in fact, unexpected information will probably be revealed.

So, why would using this information and diagnostic techniques to gather and protect personal wealth not be a positive spin off from this approach to examining our genetic makeup?

The answer, unfortunately is in the mixed messages that

society brings to the subject of money, and, the way you let those mixed messages affect your own natural strengths and weaknesses towards earning and keeping money as revealed in **The Millionaire Code.**

One of these messages is this: For many people "money isn't everything—the be all and end all of their lives." Frequently, security, a stable family life and good health are what they want.

Yet, there is a constant barrage of advertisements in virtually every media outlet designed to sell us products that improve our lives, make us look better and, in general own more than our neighbors. In fact, several popular TV car commercials actually compare the benefits of one car to the neighbor's car. Two car companies specifically target their market to one of the four financial personalities when they advertise models for those who want power, fun and control. Consumer product companies spend millions of dollars on research, testing and promotion to influence our buying habits, particularly directed at our basic personalities. The information is easily communicated, and the result is often harmful financial decisions.

Then there is the already mentioned lottery. What could send a stronger message about the value of having millions of dollars? The build up and follow up to each gigantic jackpot simply fuels the public interest and drives more people to spend money they probably could use for other, more essential things.

Of course, in order to make this message more palatable, the lottery masquerades as a charity or public service, funding education and other important causes (also the excuse used to not ban tobacco since cigarette taxes are *crucial* to state revenues). This rationale is so well accepted that only a few states do not participate in the lottery. Everywhere we look the message is you CAN have it all, and it's not hard to do so. But you have to be in it to win it. It is imbued in our culture.

Ironically, the numbers of personally wealthy millionaires have not grown in the United States. Even in an age where "millionaire" really doesn't mean what it did only 50 years ago, there is only a small percentage of the population that achieves that stature. The big picture shows that the percentage of millionaires did not increase during the late 1990s, the biggest boon period of the century. The rate remained constant at 3.5 percent of the population, fondly referred to as the 3.5 Club. Why? Throughout the period, 2.3 percent of the group (more than half of the 3.5 Club) were tracked as risky investors ready to cash out and let others cycle into club membership.

Humans fall prey to typical and predictable behavior traps; in other words, their poor behavior with money shows. So, let's face it. Between personal desires, commercial pressure, internal family issues, and just basic needs, financial decisions may not always be made with total objectivity. Your behavior/personality with money is definitely showing. What does this behavior say about you?

Medical researchers, neuroscientists and psychologists have been lecturing, writing books and even updating college textbooks with trait data gleaned from the human genome project. In 1990 Congress deemed the subsequent ten years as the "decade of the brain." Some people are catching on and buying books to match personality tests with careers and job selection. However, jobs and careers are not statistically related to staying in the 3.5 Club. Neither is race, sex, age, inheritance or education.

The bigger picture is that personality type, and inherent strengths and weaknesses are related to wealth attainment. That is the promise of **The Millionaire Code**!

The 3.5 Club

Throughout the late nineties, the IRS reported approximately 10.5 million millionaires. The US population was almost 300 million. The math is the math: 3.5% of the population had a minimum net worth (less mortgages, secured and unsecured debt) of one million dollars. Fast forward to 2002, Money Magazine reported that there were 7 million millionaires, divided by 300 million means the recession knocked 2.3% of the risky investors out of the ballpark. Statistically speaking, the 3.5 Club will return but there will always be 2.3% behaving as risky investors.

CHAPTER TWO

How The Millionaire Code Works

2

∞

Personality is the unique, limitless part of our life that makes us distinct from everyone else. It is too vast for us even to comprehend. An island in the sea may be just the top of a large mountain, and our personality is like that island. We don't know the great depths of our being.
— J. Chambers, *My Utmost for His Highest*

The Millionaire Code in each of us is actually a mental formula that identifies your money personality, lays out your strengths and weaknesses, and generally provides a framework that assesses personal wants and needs. It is based on one's genetic underpinnings, dates back thousands of years, and like other genetic DNA is needed for survival of the species. Put another way, this rubric, the initial one imprinted in man and woman that allowed them to function in an unknown world, is equally valuable in today's fast-paced, ever-changing, and truly misunderstood economy.

To help you understand this hidden code, think of this book as a roadmap to riches. First, and just like "x" marks the spot on any pirates' treasure map, you'll be asked to "x" in your answers to 16 questions. This quiz — one you'll find both entertaining and enlightening — defines anyone's relationship with money.

These sixteen questions will identify your one predominant personality code regarding financial behavior. Once you know "who you are," chapters 6-9 in the book will show you how your inherent wants relate to your personality regarding money. Then in chapters 10-12, we show you how to improve your financial status with the information.

The immediate goal is financial security with peace of mind so you have fun and control over your life. You may not be a millionaire when you finish reading this book, but one thing is sure. You'll never see money the same way, and you will know how you attract money as well as how you might push it away. Your approach to making more money and keeping it will be more methodical, clearer of purpose. That's the first step in becoming healthy, wealthy, and wise.

Final important points —

A lot of people think each person is like a snowflake, individual in *every* way. But this is not the way it is. Each person has one dominant financial personality out of four personality clusters. Think of them as the foundation of your individual snowflake. The basic ingredients for this foundation are drive, life style choices, levels of energy, extroversion or introversion, overall mood, and inherent optimism or pessimism.

Those ingredients override other demographic characteristics such as gender, race, ethnicity and family cultures. While these are not ingredients of personality, they play apart in your thoughts and behavior with money. So we have to recognize that your behavior is a result of thoughts. Thoughts, conscious or not, precede actions. Your thoughts are influenced by your sex, your ethnicity, and family background. We often *think* about and see things differently, but we can still group these responses in clusters. Your behavior is showing, and this is where your money personality can be affected.

Gender

Take "love," for example.
- Most women define love by a person's time and attention invested with them.

- Men equate love with outward indications of respect and inward content with self-esteem. This is seen clearly in the things which men and women gossip about (and by the way, men and women gossip equally, in fact, men may gossip just a bit more).
- Women gossip about their relationships and their attachments; men gossip about their achievements.

Now, take a moment and think about it. There's nothing wrong with either the male or female approach; it's just different. Both approaches are equally good. However, knowing those differences, and even striving to blend them harmoniously is a valuable tool. Ponder the concept: If two people work together instead of working at odds with each other, not only would money be saved, but marriages, too (and don't forget business relationships while we are at it). Most relationships that end cite money as a main cause.

Ethnic, Racial and Family Background

Cultural preferences regarding wealth management do impact money behavior. The positive or negative feedback we receive from our friends or family members can reinforce personality traits, either strengths or weaknesses. Too often, we only see and know ourselves by what others communicate. Our friends and family, however, are only human and assess us through their own eyes, their own personality, expectations, wants and needs. Thus, many of us need to, but never reevaluate who we are and what our financial experiences have taught us, much less return to examine our core competencies and preferences.

This is why Chambers in *My Utmost for His Highest* states that personality *"is too vast for us even to comprehend."* Jimmy Carter in *Living Faith* states that *"It is difficult for any of us to assess our own habits and actions objectively."* Rudy Giuliani reflected in an interview with *Atlanta Journal-Constitution* about leading New Yorkers through the terrorist attacks and stated that *"It* (the events of 9/11/01) *called upon different things in my personality that probably were there before."* Without new guidelines or changed situations for learning, it is not possible to know what you don't know or correct mistaken beliefs that get accepted as a way of life.

Knowing your personality is important but understanding your behavior in important relationships is a key to your thoughts. Your thoughts about money are possibly the missing link between forever struggling with money and living your dream. Changing how you think about money may be the easiest way to change your financial behavior. Except, we rarely act in total isolation.

We need to understand the people we relate to. Having a well balanced, successful relationship with good communication is part of how you can maximize the information revealed by **The Millionaire Code**. Few people really make it up the financial success ladder all alone; most don't want to. Realistically, however, some people do choose to become and remain millionaires without relationship supports, a spouse or partner. The point is that we shouldn't or usually don't lose our financial personality when we enter a relationship. However, challenges to each person's code are inherent in our differences. **The Millionaire Code** applies equally well to singles and couples.

In the subsequent chapters, we also take this relationship with money and identify how it correlates, enhances or interferes with all other relationships (regardless of gender, family background or other ethnic factors). At the heart of this entire book is that you have to look beyond the surface of your gender, race, and cultural background to what your behavior says about you and money. Why? With an unstable economy and when confronted with decisions where your money behavior may be lacking, you can harm yourself seriously and never see it coming until it's much too late.

Remember — your responses to **The Millionaire Code** profile in Chapter Three will unlock your real feelings that form your gut reaction about d̲ollars, n̲umbers and financial a̲ttitude (DNA). Based on your "Code-type," you will see the real financial you, not what others have told you. In fact, answering the 16 questions may seem humorous and tough at the same time. All four answers to each question may seem plausible, depending on different circumstances. That is the point, of course. All four behavioral approaches with money will get you secure positioning in the 3.5 Club if you lean toward strengths and don't err toward weaknesses. But, it won't help to pick what someone else thinks is the "best" answer because they have an equal number of weaknesses. If you will honestly think back over your most frequent responses to the situation at hand, only one represents you *most* of the time. That's the answer that must be "x'd" or marked in order to identify your personal strengths and weaknesses.

Accumulating wealth has everything to do with your humanness and personality strengths and weaknesses. So, do you have what it takes to set and meet your financial goals? Absolutely and we can prove it when you read on, and fill out **The Millionaire Code** profile. Just turn the page.

The Harsh Truth About Being Human

We as a nation spent a lot in the 1990s. The national savings rate plunged from 8.7 percent in 1992 to 1 percent in 2000. In addition, the average household owes 104 percent of its after-tax income (CNN/Money, 10/24/02). You know the harsh truth: We need to spend less and save more income.

Now! Discover Your Millionaire Code! The Sixteen Questions: How To Take A Quick Look At Your Results

3

∞

Instructions: Read This First!

The result of your **Millionaire Code** evaluation is only the starting point for your new, financially healthy life — or let's call it a strategy starting line. Once you complete the profile we like to say, "your behavior is showing," and you will see yourself as one of four "financial personalities."

Before you start, try to remember, once again that there are no right or wrong answers. We know, shrinks and self-help gurus always say that and a lot of times, they don't really mean it, but this time it's really true. Why? As long time research psychologists have known there are four basic personality types — not one global trait or paradigm of successful behavior, and everybody has one predominant personality type. Each personality type has strengths and weaknesses. You can "be" you and have an increased net worth of $1,000,000. You don't have to "be" someone else because they also have a list of weaknesses. So, you see, there's not one millionaire's mind, there's four, and each personality type has an equal shot at achieving their heart's and mind's desires!

Instructions

Step One: Read the questionnaire on pages 19-22. Read each question and mark the letter (**a, b, c,** or **d**) with an "X" that reminds you most of you.

Step Two: Transfer your responses (**a,b,c,** or **d**) to the answer sheet (page 24) in this book.

Step Three: Count the number of times you responded with an **a, b, c,** or **d** answer. Fill in and complete the table also on page 24.

Step Four: Once you have learned your financial personality, here's how to look at it:

The factors that make up your financial DNA are easily summed — no computer, calculator, slide-rule required. Observe and examine your highest/most frequent "score." This is your **primary behavior pattern**. The next highest count is your **blended personality pattern**. Of course, complete information on these will be fully explained in subsequent chapters.

Step Five (optional): *If* you have a significant other (designated by the letter "O" for "Other") ask them to fill out the form, repeating the steps 1-3, marking their answers with an alternative color pen and recording their totals as "O." Now one or both of you need the rest of the story!

Find Your Millionaire Code!

DIRECTIONS: Read each question and select ("X" or circle) the one answer from the four choices that sounds MOST like you, MOST of the time. There are no wrong answers, honest!

1. **When it comes to time and money,**
    a. Work to live, and live for today because tomorrow is another day.
    b. Work, work, work because time is money. Leisure can come later.
    c. Organize my life so I can find time for both work and play — what's life without a little enjoyment!
    d. Slow and steady pace wins "the race."

2. **What amount of cash do you have access to right now?**
    a. I wish I knew.
    b. Does access to credit cards and lines of credit count?
    c. I know the exact amount down to the penny.
    d. You think I'm going to tell you that? What's it to you?

3. **When it comes to long-term savings, I**
    a. Don't think about it.
    b. Wish I had money, then I would find a fast way to grow it.
    c. Save for rainy days and retirement, too.
    d. Stash plenty of cash away in savings. It's one of the things I do best.

4. **When it comes to money and happiness . . .**
    a. Money can't buy happiness, but it sure can buy a lot of fun.
    b. Money equals power; power equals happiness; therefore money equals happiness.
    c. Money can't buy me love but having money sure is warm on cold winter nights.
    d. Money buys respect and status everywhere.

5. **When it comes to personal financial responsibility . . .**
   a. If I spend more than I make, I can always make more.
   b. I *plan* to earn big and save big but often spend big.
   c. I work very hard to live and spend within my means.
   d. It's very important to financially help family in trouble.

6. **When I have left-over money after all the bills are paid, I**
   a. Spend it immediately.
   b. Save or invest a little, but spend most of it.
   c. Save or invest most of it, but spend a little.
   d. Save or invest all of it.

7. **Dollars and numbers, how are you with details?**
   a. I hate payment schedules and deadlines involved in handling money.
   b. I love numbers but hate it when dollars/investments don't perform as planned.
   c. I design detailed budgets and hate it when I have to deviate from my plan.
   d. I use a wait and watch approach to handling dollars, numbers, and I hate *having* to take action.

8. **When it comes to shopping,**
   a. I shop, therefore I buy.
   b. I plan, stay up on prices, then shop, in and out fast.
   c. I organize, and then I buy.
   d. I need a lifestyle similar to my friends, and then I buy to match it.

9. **When it comes to sales . . .**
   a. Sale — it's the most beautiful word in the whole-wide world.
   b. Finding a great deal is the 2nd best thing in the world.
   c. I shop sales — brand names usually — but I get buyer's remorse a lot and return them.
   d. I love shopping warehouses or specialty stores that sell limited, quality merchandise inexpensively.

10. **When it comes to monthly money management,**
   a. It's a lot like playing Monopoly.
   b. I prefer to make the decisions about how money is spent.
   c. I need to handle it just right, even perfectly; if I think I can't, I will pass the torch.
   d. I manage it the easy way: deposit it and forget I have it.

11. **When it comes to my being without funds . . .**
   a. Being broke is the second or third worst thing that could happen to me.
   b. As long as I've got good credit available, I can rebuild and create growth.
   c. Being flat broke is the worst thing that can happen to me.
   d. Being broke is failure, and it must be avoided at all costs.

12. **What's the best way to achieve financial security?**
   a. Get creative, work with lots of good people, produce and serve others.
   b. Take charge and control your own destiny.
   c. Watch the details, analyze choices, and make calculated decisions.
   d. Find a niche and fill it up. Be the guru.

13. **How much money is enough money?**
   a. Why set limits? This is a land of opportunity.
   b. Enough to spring-board and try more money-making possibilities.
   c. 20% more than I make now.
   d. Enough to guarantee comfort and peace of mind.

14. **How do you respond to financial stress?**
    a. Easily distracted, worried, anxious, sleep less, experience heart palpitations, and have a short fuse.
    b. Grow more headstrong and critical, sometimes heartburn, stomach burning, hot/cold flashes.
    c. Get moody and withdraw, oversleep, overeat, along with muscle or joint pains or digestive problems.
    d. Doubtful, indecisive, sluggish, procrastinate and congestion gets worse (allergies, sinus, or asthma).

15. **Which money motto fits your buying style?**
    a. Only one more shopping day until tomorrow!
    b. Spend money my way!
    c. You get what you pay for!
    d. Peace at any price!

16. **When it comes to financial planning...**
    a. Help!
    b. Just do it!
    c. I do it, and it is only fair that others do their part too.
    d. I'll get around to it.

Interpretation:

As we've just mentioned, after you finish the questionnaire, mark your answers on the following answer sheet in this book for reference later, either a, b, c, d as shown on the answer sheet. It is a good idea to repeat this exercise annually to re-evaluate your behavior with dollars, numbers and attitude about money-conscious behaviors. It is unlikely that we use all our available strengths at one time. Some strengths are more accessible with changing relationship demands, health status, different ages and stages. We can more easily meet goals and expectations when our inherent weaknesses are minimized or irrelevant to any problem at hand and our inherent strengths meet the particular need at the time.

Again, add up and total each of your a, b, c and d answers.

The letter you chose most frequently reveals your **primary Millionaire Code** of behavior:

(a) Pleasure Seeker

(b) Powerbroker

(c) Problem Solver

(d) Peacemaker.

The higher number of the same letter above means you are more likely to fit that "personality DNA" where money is concerned.

For example, if your highest count was 8 "b" answers, Powerbroker is your predominant approach.

If your next highest score was 5 "a" answers, you are a blend of Powerbroker (primarily) and Pleasure Seeker (secondarily). It is possible and even likely that you will have high scores in more than one category. After all, you are unique but typically a blending of two DNA approaches with money.

So what? What do your answers mean? It means your behavior is showing; you can predict your money behavior pattern; and it means we can help you choose your next financial course of action. Then you will be able to take charge, have fun, security and peace of mind. Read on to learn your strengths and weaknesses. Then it is up to you to use your personal **Millionaire Code.**

YOUR MILLIONAIRE CODE DATA REPORT

THE MILLIONAIRE CODE	TOTAL #A-D ANSWERS FOR YOU				TOTAL #A-D ANSWERS FROM OTHER			
DNA TEST QUESTION#	A	B	C	D	A	B	C	D
1. "When it comes to time…"								
2. "What amount of cash do…"								
3. "When it comes to long-term…"								
4. "When it comes to money…"								
5. "When it comes to personal…"								
6. "When I have left-over money…"								
7. "Dollars and numbers, the…"								
8. "When it comes to shopping…"								
9. "When it comes to sales…"								
10. "When it comes to monthly…"								
11. "When it comes to being…"								
12. "What's the best way to…"								
13. "How much money is enough…"								
14. "How do you respond to stress…"								
15. "Which money motto fits…"								
16. "When it comes to financial…"								
Total # Xs in each column								

Total # "a" responses	Total # "b" responses	Total # "c" responses	Total # "d" responses
____ / ____ You/Other	____ / ____ You/Other	____ / ____ You/Other	____ / ____ You/Other
Pleasure Seeker	Powerbroker	Problem Solver	Peacemaker
Money means more fun, love, and we can live it up today!	Money means power, self worth, control.	Money means security, clear conscience.	Money means peace of mind, respect, financial status

A Visual Way To See Your Status

Now, let's take a picture of your answers. First we'll graph a sample set of typical personality types below and then you put your own total scores on the next graph, page 28. This might be "typical" raw scores for two partners.

Financial Personality Data Chart

X = YOU   **O = OTHER**

SCORES	A = Pleasure Seeker	B = Power-broker	C = Problem Solver	D = Peace-maker
16				
15				
14				
13				
12				
11				
10	X		O	
9				
8				
7				
6				O
5				
4		X		
3				
2			X	
1				
0	O	O		X

Summary of Example Scores:

Total # "a" responses	Total # "b" responses	Total # "c" responses	Total # "d" responses
10 / 0	4 / 0	2 / 10	0 / 6
You (X)/(O)Other	You (X)/(O)Other	You (X)/(O)Other	You (X)/(O)Other
Pleasure Seeker	Powerbroker	Problem Solver	Peacemaker

In the above graph, we see two people who are opposite financial personalities. **"Person X"** is extroverted with highest scores on "a" and "b" answers. **"Person O"** is introverted with highest scores for "c" and "d" answers.

"X" has a high score on Pleasure Seeker with money and a blended, secondary score on Powerbroker. X will be good at exploring ways to create wealth. **"O"** on the other hand, is not an adventurer with money. O has a low score on Pleasure Seeker and on Powerbroker but a high primary score on Problem Solver blended with Peacemaker.

Person O (Spouse or Partner), in this example, will be excellent with details, numbers and tightly managing dollars. They are often referred to as "genius" when educated about money. They are the best to manage the checkbook. They will have a very realistic, but sometimes pessimistic, attitude about managing financial wealth.

According to the above hypothetical analysis, **Person X,** being primarily a Pleasure Seeker, will be completely optimistic with money, possibly to the point of being a spend-a-holic. These people should *not ordinarily* handle the checkbook but need a role in wealth management. They are naturally good shoppers and have a good eye for price, quantity, quality and sales. If they are educated about finances, they can be creative shoppers for investments, either real estate or bond and stock markets. They might even recognize great values when those markets go on sale, as they usually do, about every seven years.

Their low score on problem solving, however, means they won't appreciate the details and time it takes to shore up wealth management. These are mainstay concepts for **Person O** in our example. Problem Solvers naturally value the details when given sufficient time. In summary, this relationship will be divisive over money at times and will need to rely on good communication while allowing each to develop their individual wealth building skills. You can see how valuable **The Millionaire Code** can be for the example relationship.

Now, how about you? Whether you are a single person or you two are a duo, what are your strengths and weaknesses? Transfer your own total counts of **a, b, c, d** scores to the following table.

Total # "a" responses	Total # "b" responses	Total # "c" responses	Total # "d" responses
_____/_____	_____/_____	_____/_____	_____/_____
(X)/(O)	**(X)/(O)**	**(X)/(O)**	**(X)/(O)**
Pleasure Seeker	Powerbroker	Problem Solver	Peacemaker

To transfer scores to graph, **YOU** can mark an X parallel to each score in a, b, c, and d blocks. **O** can use dots instead of Xs. Connect the Xs or Os and note the differences.

SCORES	A = Pleasure Seeker	B = Power-broker	C = Problem Solver	D = Peace-maker
16				
15				
14				
13				
12				
11				
10				
9				
8				
7				
6				
5				
4				
3				
2				
1				
0				

Pleasure Seeker   Powerbroker   Problem Solver   Peacemaker

Take time for your own "Aha" experience. At this point, we've seen people come alive and wake up to the fact that they can be wealthy if they will just get out of their own way.

CHAPTER FOUR

Why This Works

4
∞

Congratulations! You just passed a "test" you cannot fail. Now what you do with this clear-cut, simple knowledge can change your life. Odd, isn't it? Unlocking your financial personality and analyzing your behavior with money seems to be common sense. Yet millions of people have gone lifetimes never knowing and understanding why they do what they do, for better or worse. The information is far more than a neat-and-clean label. Used correctly, it can introduce you to your financial strengths and weaknesses, security, and perhaps wealth. That is why the rest of this book is devoted to a step-by-step, tried-and-true strategy; one that will help you unlock your **Millionaire Code**.

Step One: Understand personality and why it's so powerful.

Step Two: Appreciate and lean toward your specific, inherent strengths.

Step Three: Confront your weaknesses. Why? Because the good news is that any weakness, any behavior that doesn't contribute to your goals, any behavior you don't like can be overridden with new brain software. Every journey starts with hope and a first step, and that step is neurochemically locked away inside your own head.

As deceptively simple as it sounds, your brain biology affects your handing of money. Like all emotions, there are neurochemicals, along with biological DNA, which come together to create money personality. In fact, today's scientists believe that our brains are more hardwired at birth than previously thought, and that's a good thing. It allows us to approach some of life in an almost routine, automatic fashion. If that were not the case, even the brightest among us would be overwhelmed by the exigencies and vicissitudes of life. As a result, most of what seems automatic and normal behavior is the result of hardwired, genetic predispositions that have been intact for as long as there has been functioning on this planet. Your parents not only gave you the gift of life, they gave you the gift of one of four predominant personalities which, by the way, may not be necessarily just like either of them.

Here's a hardwired example straight out of the "Pleasure Seeker" and "Powerbroker" arsenal of behaviors. Researchers have made progress and linked novelty seeking (a primary trait for the Pleasure Seeker) with a gene that produces the protein responsible for creating a dopamine receptor called DRD4. Fancy words that mean a little spendthrift thrill may be the result of the push of a brain chemical.

Here's a hardwired example for the "Problem Solver" and "Peacemaker." They have an inherent need to check and double check. They may even do the same behaviors over and over when that action has been less than effective due to a "shot" of "brain juice" called serotonin (technically it's a serotonin transporter gene or 5-HTTLPR). In straightforward terms, there is plenty of scientific evidence that personality tendencies have a genetic component and influence brain responses.

Does this mean behavior is totally predetermined? To some degree, "yes," and to some degree, "no." That's not meant to sound like double talk; there's just a great deal about the brain that researchers don't understand yet. What does appear incontrovertible and abundantly clear is that you have a pre-wired system in place, a starting point. It's one that you can always rely on, but your incoming thoughts turn genes "on" and "off" depending on your needs at a given time. In stressful situations, you may turn "off" new learning and turn "on" old behaviors that feel good (psychologists call that "spontaneous regression"); new learning takes a back seat. These old behaviors may not solve the problem; it's just that working in our weaknesses feels better, more secure. This explains why many people, when stressed to the max with the lack of money, allow their old personality code — one that got them into trouble to begin with — to "rescue" them.

Behavior is NOT totally predetermined. You always have a choice. Humans are not predestined to wallow in poverty or squander millions. While genes sometimes seem to stand firm like the Rock of Gibraltar, our thoughts can turn genes "on" and "off."

> Your brain has always responded to sensory rewards but the latest brain research shows that it perks up at the prospect of monetary ones. The reward circuit runs on the neurochemical dopamine. Economic Nobelists are 2002 winners because they recognize that economic decisions, like all others, reflect brain activity. Some people seem wired to delay immediate gratification of profit in the stock market and some go for broke.
>
> (Begley, Sciencejournal@wsj.com, 11/15/02)

Genes are little biochemical recipes, and as you pass through life, you're allowed to season to taste. Overall, genes are not an instruction for action; they are a set point, a default code when all else fails. You may be pre-wired; you may not think you have control, but you are free to choose thoughts and behaviors. In fact, the conscious brain has a built in veto power, an out-clause, and the function is identical to a mental computer questioning, "Are you sure?" Even after you make a conscious, volitional decision to act, there's a 100-200-millisecond period where your brain asks you to re-evaluate the decision you've made. It's like your brain's saying, "Are you sure you want to do what your gene recipe is demanding?"

The Wall Street Science Journal recently reported a case where thoughts literally turned genes on. A report in the *Journal* described a scientist spending several weeks studying on a remote island in comparative isolation. The day before he was due for shore leave, he experienced a flood of testosterone anticipating the resumption of sexual activity. Physically, he even experienced a noticeable growth in his beard. This man's *"thought-ful"* experience demonstrated what multiple studies about thoughts and concomitant responses have shown.

Brain biology is shaped by genetic connections, but it is imprinted by sensory systems (i.e., touch, taste, sight, pain, and temperature) throughout our life. Unlike many organs that start out small and grow big, the brain starts out big but grows smaller. In the first 45 days of life, the brain quadruples its connections. But between the ages of 3 and 15 years, we lose billions of those carefully forged synaptic connections. By the age of 16, half of the network is gone, and by 20 years of age the code is in place — it may not be perfect, but it's a complete daily operation manual.

Routine behavior is primarily a response to gene instruction. Remember, it's a gene recipe that days, weeks, months, and years have seasoned to taste. Over time, these genes instructed nerve cells to branch out, much like a tree (about ten thousand connections or synapses with other nerve cells). As a result, personality solidifies over time primarily from initial, code-like genetic communication. The environment influences the communication and the family/environmental "thought" message is increasingly recognized as a critical factor that changes the brain by altering its connections.

What does this mean about your behavior with money? Personality, early-life experiences, current stress (good and bad), health, and age status contribute to gene instruction that ultimately expresses itself as behavior with money. Just like your computer, your system will default to its pre-wired money operating system (MOS) unless you change the instruction and do something specific to focus on your strengths. That's okay if you're satisfied with your financial wealth building. But, if not, you have a choice. Here's the code-building or code-unlocking choice:

(1) Do nothing and your pre-wired system will take over. It will search for the easiest and often the weakest link to implement;

(2) Add new, more powerful software that overrides any pre-wired personality system that's causing all the problems.

Berating ourselves and leaning toward our weaknesses are easier than focusing on building strengths. Across all cultures, surveyors for the Gallup Poll reported that the only age group that positively acknowledged and consistently focused on strengths was the elder population. Why wait until then? There is no reason. Re-evaluating life experiences and personality strengths with money is important, now and reevaluate again later. The rest of the book will help you do just that.

Now you know your code's name — either Pleasure Seeker, Powerbroker, Problem Solver, or Peacemaker. You know where it came from and it's time to learn its strengths and weaknesses, and bring your current brain code kicking and screaming into the 21st Century. Not to worry, your brain will get the idea soon enough that you're not changing out of one code into another. You're just taking charge, control of some of its power for the better.

HOW DOES YOUR ANNUAL EXPENSES STACK UP TO THE AVERAGE HOUSEHOLD EXPENDITURES (AFTER FEDERAL, STATE, SOCIAL SECURITY TAXES)?

Housing	33%
Transportation	20% (purchases, leases, rentals, maintenance, gas)
Healthcare, incidentals	18%
Food, dining in/out	14%
Childcare	10% (grandparents not exempt)
Vacations, holidays, movies	5%

Source: Money/CNN, 10/24/02

How You Attract Money & How You Push It Away

PERSONALITY	HOW DO YOU ATTRACT MONEY?	PUSH IT AWAY?
Pleasure Seeker (Money = love, fun)	• the spirited promoter leads the charge. • they network and enlist others' help. • they shop the alternatives and pick wisely. • they "see" the big picture. • they plan for sunny days. • they earn by teaching, selling, talking,and promoting. • money is way of expressing love. . .	• they stay uneducated. • they delegate *all* and remain uninvolved. • they limit advice by choosing to work with others *just* like them. • they don't see details. • don't plan for rainy days. • they lose by not listening and hearing. • but money can be used for self-aggrandizement.
Powerbroker (Money = power and control)	• they earn by making correct decisions fast. • they get the big picture... • they delegate... • they compete; ... • they exert power and control,. . .	• every situation is not correctly solved with a fast answer. • then give up control. • and devalue the details. • then forget to cooperate. • but don't control self.
Problem Solver (Money = self esteem & security)	• they study, order, and care to organize. • they resolve problems, handle details. • schedule and balance money, lifestyle. • pursues doing things the right way. • self-esteem means self-respect...	• any uncertainty is depressing. • details are huge burdens. • "right way" *always* is expressway to stress way! • or self-conceit?
Peacemaker (Money = peace of mind, clear conscious)	• they earn by being highly educated, a respected guru. • patient and competent savers! • generous and helps others.	• loses when chooses to ignore big picture. • managers, not leaders • loans money but rarely paid back and can't afford to forfeit.

If You Live By Your Weaknesses, Salesmen Love You!

5

∞

Whether its office supplies, clothes, cars, life insurance, real estate, or high-ticket electronic gadgets, sales agents know a lot about personality. What does your financial personality tell them when it comes to taking your money?

Pleasure Seekers leaning toward their weaknesses are nicknamed "the puppet" for the easy way salesmen pull your strings. The Pleasure Seeker responds in kind and displays their potentially self-absorbed, self-indulgent, and egotistical behaviors. For example, salesmen play to your need to tell stories, be loved and have fun. They get Pleasure Seekers to lean back and tell the salesman a story about how smart and successful they are. The salesman *understands* that you need a "special" package, walks away — usually to talk with the sales manager — and comes back with a standard package geared to please. Their goal is to spark a friendship because that is what you communicate about wants and needs. The Pleasure Seeker thinks the salesman is their friend!

The Pleasure Seeker tends to stay on the fun track, optimistic on finding the "magic bullet" for millionaire status. Clients have even referred to themselves as "swingers" with investments because they want to catch the ascension and avoid the descent. Unfortunately, they can lose big trying to time the market as well as overlooking costs related to commissions and tax ramifications.

Powerbrokers leaning toward weaknesses are nicknamed "the boss" for their potential to direct, domineer, and "call the shots." Salesmen make observations about Powerbroker's firm (even a bit painful) handshake, rapid-fire, staccato-voice inflections and any other communications about the essence of time.

Then, they ask Powerbrokers up front how much time they can have to directly meet their need. When Powerbrokers typically say 10 minutes, they ask you if you would rather have a proposal or sales document in writing. Yes to either is the magic answer; they have the "razzle-dazzle" ready on return presentation, ready to capture your dollars.

The Powerbroker is on the fast track, but when working toward weaknesses, they can be on the verge of a multi-vessel heart bypass. They optimistically pursue a fast search for a new road to riches. Clients have even referred to themselves as "scalpers" on investments. Obviously, by using the term they see themselves as buying and selling so as to make small quick profits or to profit by slight market fluctuations. One other definition of scalpers, however, is "to remove an upper or better part." In this case, that *better part* might refer to the better part of long-term profits, for example, compounded interest and dividends inherent in well-thought out, good financial investments.

Problem Solvers leaning toward their weaknesses are known as the "questioner" for the potential to mistrust, doubt, and subject everything to analysis, interrogation. Salesmen hate to see you walk in the door, and that's not all bad. Salesmen evaluate introverted signs of behavior, the skeptical smile, ambivalent handshake and/or few words. If sized up to be introverted, they look for differences between the perfectionist Problem Solver and the Peacemaker. The perfectionist asks so many questions, and offers "yes, but" enough that they salesman won't spend too much time on you — you are too boring, too hesitant — too much trouble and you won't buy anyway.

The Problem Solver tends to search for *the perfect* path to a balanced financial status. With financial advisors, they even refer to themselves as "the bargain shopper" when it comes to investments. Certainly, bargains can be had, but timing is important and these people do not appreciate deadlines. Instead of being energized by details when it comes to money, they lean toward weaknesses and are burdened with details, the charts, tables, gross, net profits. They turn pessimistic with any communication that resembles hype. Most are still analyzing the investment that gained 400% *last year*. Relocate your **Millionaire Code** and join the 3.5 Club.

Peacemakers can flip to weaknesses at the sight of a sales pitch and are nicknamed "lapdog" for the potential to be molded and to make peace with the salesman. Peacemakers will not confront or negotiate. They have no desire to be antagonistic and will go out of their way to keep the peace and avoid any semblance of disrespect. Peacemakers will (accidentally but freely) pay more if you promise not to question them or challenge them in any way. Salesmen read the tea leaves; and if it looks as if you're not going to buy, they act impatient, abrupt or even angry. Now, you'll pay more just to keep the salesman calm.

Additionally, the Peacemaker tends to choose the easiest path with finances because they intend to preserve a clear conscious. We have heard them describe their personal approach to financial investments as "followers of the big boys." Investment advisors love this information because they think they are the big boys. They have *the* solution and followers are the ideal clients. However, timing and monitoring your investments to meet your goals is part of your responsibility. Being a follower typically means you follow along *behind* the profits of the big boys. Use your **Millionaire Code** to step out in front with personal strengths.

Which path would you take? Would you take the path associated with your strengths, perhaps the road less traveled; or would you default and just do it like you've done it so many times before? In the next four chapters, these four personality types are fully explained. Then the subsequent two chapters will explain how both blended personalities and conflicting partner personality weaknesses can be overcome.

Lean toward your strengths! Profit from them! Lean toward your weaknesses, and you'll continually wonder "what went wrong?" Read and refer to the chart that follows as you learn how to maximize your strengths and unlock your financial personality in the following chapters.

COMPARE YOUR DNA (Dollars, Numbers Attitude)
TRAITS, STRENGTHS, AND WEAKNESSES

YOUR CODE	TRAITS	DNA STRENGTHS	DNA WEAKNESSES
PLEASURE SEEKERS	• Playful. • Now Oriented. • Talkative. • Life of the Party. • Believe in Good. • Full of energy. • Forgiving nature. • Make Friends. • Curious. • Bored by Routine. • Imaginative. • Spontaneous. • Extroverted.	• Uses money to truly express love for others. • Generous. • Let's go (anywhere, everywhere) ...and spend money! • Money = Fun • No Pressure! I'll buy it! • Fast Paced, Fun Lovers, • Storytellers, Disney-files • Spend it now! • No illusions about money — • Can't take it with you! • Shops Sales • Finds Best Deals • Needs Money for parties, clothes, & entertaining. • Easily swayed • Open to all recommendations. • Today oriented.	• Spend it NOW! • Can't take it with you. • No money = No fun. • Feels unloved and unlovable without $$. • Flighty, distracted, sleeps less, worried under $ stress with anxiety and heart palpitations. • Overlooks plans for tomorrow. • Spend thrift behavior. • Prone to high-risk investments. • Loses Track of Facts. • "Why am I out of money if I still have checks in my check-book?" • Mark for many a con scheme. • May even keep on spending when they know they must stop. • When confronted, lies. • Never takes into account all costs

YOUR CODE	TRAITS	DNA STRENGTHS	DNA WEAKNESSES
POWER-BROKERS	• Inventive • Passionate • Assertive • Needs approval. • Strong willed • In control • Efficient • Productive • Tactless • Quarrelsome • Not into Art • Extroverted • Change-agent	• "I am the best person to control money" • Goal oriented, tight schedules. • Acts on the fast track • Money is for power • Money is for self-control • Pound wise (but penny foolish) • Spend it — can always make more. • See it my way (we stay friends). • Prefers competition to cooperation. • Not afraid of change or chaos • Goals are comprehensive, measurable	• Intimidates Others with Money On alert to get rich quick and go for broke. • Demanding, is so sure as to cram financial decisions down others throats. • Focuses on "I win-you lose". • Timetable not reasonable • Headstrong & critical • Attacks & distracts • Tends to have heartburn, hot flashes, stomach acid, ulcers, & strokes. • Charge it! Make it up next month.
PROBLEM SOLVERS	• Analytical • Considerate • Kind • Tactful • Deep Thinker • Ingenious • Unselfish • Helpful • Reliable • Keeps tight schedule. • Art/music Sophisticate. • Fault Finder. • Easily Saddened. • Introverted	• Genius thinkers • Organized planners • Slow to take action • Patiently searches for the one right investment. • Keep money thoughts to themselves/locked away. • Wants only the RIGHT way • Not easily pushed around except among safe havens • Open to secure, safe havens • Never met a money problem they couldn't solve (unless it is two+ intricately meshed problems). • Wants facts, details, good with charts and tables, projections, analysis of dollars, numbers.	• THE Right way is excruciatingly security-conscious • Gets sucked into financial ruts • Flat Broke = Worst Thing Ever • If they don't think they can perform perfectly, they don't act. • Under stress, oversleeps, overeats, moody, fussy, judgmental, withdrawn, digestion and joint aches/problems. • Too often closed to compromise • Aversive to chaos. • Very fearful of anything that is not a sure thing. • Suffers from Buyer's Remorse • Loses all emotional cool when security is threatened

YOUR CODE	TRAITS	DNA STRENGTHS	DNA WEAKNESSES
PEACE-MAKERS	• Watchful • Patient • Dry Sense of Humor • Relaxed • No Decision Maker • Good Listener • Cooperator • Compromiser • Indecisive • Quiet & Aloof • Shy • Introverted • Mediator	• Always finds the Easy Way Out • Keep the peace is the most important thing of all. Peace of mind is their mission in life. • Patient! • Money is for financial status. • Open to Cooperation. • Slow and steady reaps rewards. • Go along, don't rock the boat. • Happiest when money is placed in safe havens. • Wants to see money grow. • Clarity of purpose: • Save for a rainy day • Guru in chosen financial areas. • Usually ready, willing to help family in need. • Maintains status quo. • Good management skills.	• Can be careless, indifferent, worried under financial stress, e.g., shaky, congested, exhausted, • Sluggish, fearful, mumbles, bored, doubtful, indecisive. • Closed to competition. • Not willing to compromise when family wants adventure, fun. • Lazy with money. • Avoids change, responsibility. • Throws Money at Problems to keep the peace (e.g., his children in a divorce/tries to buy them off) • No money help wanted or needed. • Either stingy or unselfish, no in between • Risk is a four-letter fear word • May hide money where spouse can't find it or to hurt others.

Millionaire Code Stories

Andrew prefers to be a creative Peacemaker, but he can get tough, especially with salesmen when he turns it into a creative game. Take car purchases for instance. This man can buy a car better than anyone. Here's his simple strategy. He just deflects the pressure from himself back onto the salesperson and car dealership, where the pressure should be. They're always ready to see him leave, and typically give him a too-good-so sweet deal just to get him out of the dealership. Here's how it works.

Peacemaker takes over first, and he goes in as a mild-mannered car shopper. That's the first hour. After they think he's an easy emotional mark, a "lapdog" — one so easy to work with, he'll just buy and not think — then the Problem Solver kicks in and his mission, "To wear them down first. My ace in the hole is that I know the wholesale price plus roll backs on the car going in, and then I keep a running list of all their offers. Car dealers hate this. They prefer to give you an offer, take it away, and then come back with new numbers just to confuse you." In fact, he's been known to take up to 5 hours to negotiate a car. "And I always go in near the end of the month, and late in the day. Say round four o'clock, and I know they close at ten, so the closer to ten it gets, instead of their being in control, I'm in the driver's seat, pun intended. And it's fun to beat sales people at their own game. All you have to say to them, is 'No, ain't gonna do that, and stick to your guns.'" Also, when it comes time to deal with checking the final numbers, he takes out his calculator and verifies everything against his running list of prices. He says, "It's not unusual to find that they've added $500 worth of errors, stuff you never agreed to on the final invoice — something that people rarely check."

What's the moral of the story? Look out for lapdogs in questioner clothing, otherwise appreciated as the Peacemaker in problem solving attire. Acknowledge and address your personality flaws.

Current affairs

No one financial personality is immune to greed and immoral temptations. Any of the four **Millionaire Codes** are subject to taking their strengths to extreme and exercising weaknesses. Current corporate behavior including lack of morality, however, extends beyond personality weaknesses. Leaning toward weaknesses is costly! But giving in to immoral or scandalous behaviors is potentially off the scale in costs.

Are you "mad about money?" Ashley is furious and shared her thoughts.

Look no further than the scandals of 'book-cooking' by all these public companies and their public accounting firms to see that money was a motivator for a lot of lying and stealing which resulted in thousands of people being hurt financially. What was it about having all that extra money at the expense of others that would motivate the guilty parties to do what they did? Did they want to buy more stuff? Did they want to prove they were smarter than they really were by pretending the companies were doing better than they were?

Did they think they could get away with it and then just leave the company with their millions while their successor took the fall? If you look at the root motivating cause for almost every crime, scandal, or business decision, it almost always comes down to money. Whenever anybody asks, "Why in the world would someone do something like that?" Follow the money, and you'll find your answer. The greed and absolute lack of morals displayed by these people is astounding. It makes me embarrassed to be in advertising. I feel like I am responsible for contributing to people desiring things they don't want or need. But then there are other people who are exposed to advertising, and they seem to be able to control themselves. Okay, I'll get off my soapbox now.

Character is what you choose to do with your personality.

CHAPTER SIX

The Peacemaker: Easy Does It

6

∞

To say that Peacemakers are financially reserved is an under-statement. As a result, they're sure–footed, full of patience, adapt-able and so easily satisfied! It doesn't take a lot of money to make them happy. They do not aggressively seek money — they're perfectly content to have it fall into their lap. They can watch their money or other people's money and derive pleasure either way. One of their biggest joys in life is watching other people spend anybody's money except theirs!

In a credit card, pay it on-line culture, they still use the green stuff. For them, cash makes the world go round and simplifies their life. When they invest, they put the money where it will keep the peace and avoid negative confrontation. It's not unusual to find a stash of cash under their mattress. Why? It helps them sleep better at night. To take it a step further, if the money is not tied up in a safe certificate of deposit or buried in the backyard, they are usually willing to help out family members. It's not unusual to find them assisting in financing healthcare or housing, co-signing loans, and picking up checks in restaurants — after all, it helps the family and most importantly of all, it keeps the peace.

> Circlelending.com is reporting that more than 7 million
> person-to-person loans are outstanding among friends, rela-
> tives and peers at any given time. The amount represents over
> 4% of the $1.5 trillion consumer credit market (11/18/02). If
> you choose to loan, draw up a contract for repayment or
> consider gifting the money.

To prove that "keeping the peace is their reason for being," they typically enable family members to overspend and to take risks. They'll do anything to avoid a confrontation or saying, "No." Granted, most of us can identify with the need to keep the peace in families, but these individuals take it to the extreme. Their DNA financial personality motivates them to invest in peace even if it has few even no financial returns. We mean this literally. They often do not pursue reimbursement for family loans. If the borrower does not offer to pay debts back, the Peacemaker will likely "let sleeping dogs lie." They do without rather than making demands.

Just as Sherlock Holmes had Moriarty, Peacemakers have a nemesis, too. Spending money, shopping, can be an adversarial process. It is hard work and takes way too much energy. Shopping with Peacemakers is a slow and steady experience, not necessarily fun like the Pleasure Seeker would have it; certainly not right on the money as preferred by the Problem Solver; and definitely not fast like the Powerbroker demands. Because shopping around is hard work, they tend to purchase items from specialty or small stores. They will make repetitive visits to stores that provide good but limited choices. While they are forever looking for and bragging about bargains, they are not good at shopping for them, so they often look, but don't purchase anything on sale. To add insult to injury, when they do "break down" and spend, any amount of money is too much. Then, because they're "cheapskates," buyer's remorse kicks in. But don't confuse these cheapskates with pleasure seeking bargain hunters who flock to malls on bargain days after Christmas or Thanksgiving. This behavior is conspicuously absent. The festive, frenetic, joyous hoopla just exacerbates their acid stomach tendencies.

Since they're naturally laid back, overly relaxed, chilled beyond belief, the persistent Peacemaker devalues tension. Our DNA financial trait data identifies them as inherently consistent with money, patient, calm, cool, and collected, and routinely slowed down by inertia! They are a balancing act, struggling to balance being happily reconciled to life and needing the self-motivation to ensure the future of that happiness. That's why they avoid money responsibility and are lazy with personal budgets. While teenagers respond to competing points of view with "whatever," Peacemakers simply say, "I'll worry about it later in life." But . . .they never do.

When they hit the "Big 5-0", or any big birthday for that matter, inertia keeps them on the same path. Change is tough for this personality: change equals trouble or at least problems; and problems require action, maybe even new responsibilities. Age 50+ is SO hard if they aren't financially prepared. If Murphy's Law kicks in — and it usually does at least once or twice in a given lifetime — they fall back on old Peacemaker habits, the same ones that didn't work the last time.

What is Murphy's Law? It is one of the most famous eponyms — the legacy of one very picky Air Force officer. In the late 1940s, Capt. Ed Murphy, an aircraft engineer by training, complained about an incompetent technician on his team. "If there is any way to do it wrong, he will," Murphy said. His co-workers began calling the captain's pessimism Murphy's Law, and mentioned it in a press conference. As long as people keep on making mistakes, Murphy will live (*Reader's Digest*, Dec. 2001, pg. 132).

Here are examples of Peacemaker DNA in the real world.

Peacemaker Millionaire DNA Personality #1: Jimmy Carter, 39th President of the United States, Nobel Peace Prize Laureate, Fall 2002

Former President James Earl Carter Jr. is one of the world's most respected Peacemakers, and he's got the financial DNA to prove it. However, since most of us are blended personalities, we believe he is a Peacemaker when it comes to money, but Carter's work behavior is more typical of Problem Solvers. For instance, as President, the perfectionist Problem Solver in him thrived on details, schedules and discipline with clearly defined priorities and a known pace. When he assumed the presidency, the press summarized his strengths: Strong moral compass, self-confident, amazing self-discipline, detailed knowledge of major issues, refusal to compromise his standards, and appeal as an honest outsider. All of these qualify as strengths for Problem Solvers.

But by the third year of his presidency, his abilities were taxed; his strengths were taken to extremes and flipped to weaknesses. He bounced from working within his strengths, defaulted, and relied on tried-and-true comfortable behaviors that just didn't work. Now the press described him as aimless, drifting, remote, losing touch, depressed and frightened. *Newsweek* reported that *"Jimmy Carter appears to have been a hard man to work for–demanding, highly critical of inadequate staff work, yet rarely complimentary of a good job."* Over-analysis quickly became paralysis, common for perfect Problem Solvers.

Where money and finances were concerned, however, we observed more behaviors in keeping with Peacemakers. Remember, Peacemakers do not value money in the same way other personalities do. Financial status is important, of course, as well as keeping the peace, and there is everything right and nothing wrong with that. But strengths are intricately tied to weaknesses, and financial Peacemakers tend to avoid taking charge of making changes where money is concerned — even when change is desperately needed. Sometimes inactivity is the right activity. However, too much of anything such as indecision and inactivity can be a bad thing. For instance, interest rates remained at an all time high for a protracted period of time during Carter's administration, inflation increased, recession continued and fuel shortages worsened. Peacemakers prefer to watch monetary trends (and watch and watch and watch).

Carter's 1996 autobiography, *Living Faith*, reflects the serious and purposeful emotions of a Peacemaker personality. We especially appreciated and understood how he summarized his rules of thought — abstracted as follows.

1. Peacemakers do not break rules. They follow them to the letter!
2. Peacemakers have a *dry* sense of humor, …*always* based on truth that often surprises people. A preacher once asked

President Carter how he could be a Christian, a deacon and a Sunday school teacher *and* become involved in politics? He gave him a wonderfully accurate, but terse response: "I will have 75,000 people in my senate district. How would you like to have a congregation that big?"

3. Peacemakers believe, as President Carter states, "...differences among groups of people sap a tremendous portion of our ability, time, money and influence" only to result in "internecine warfare, in arguments and debates that not only are divisive but incapacitate us for our work." For the Peacemaker, diplomacy, tolerance, adaptability are highly valued characteristics. Differences worth arguing about unfortunately bring challenge and challenge means problems and problems *should* be addressed slowly. Change is not always right or good. So they prefer to watch, ...wait patiently.

4. Peacemakers enjoy "lively debate but (with) few injured feelings." They are sensitive and thoughtful listeners on topics of interest. They prefer to zero in and learn a lot about specific issues in order to be the "guru" in those areas.

But those pesky Peacemaker weaknesses were always apparent. He admitted that for the first seven years of marriage, he and his wife, Rosalyn, just watched their money, not saving except a little in a few war bonds (a very conservative investment). Watching money can be a pastime for Peacemakers. Peacemakers are also excellent listeners but usually don't speak until they are perfectly sure of what to say. In *Living Faith*, he admitted he was often silent or uncommunicative. When Rosalyn expressed concern that he was displeased with her or was falling out of love, the Peacemaker admitted becoming angry and even more withdrawn.

Consciousness of personality traits precedes good communication and the young Peacemaker said he was unaware of what caused so much discomfort. In typical Peacemaker fashion, communication weaknesses, such as not *"telling it like it is"* followed by long silences, can have huge negative consequences — in business, marriages, and parenting relationships. The Carters' love for each other prevailed even though he continued to fall prey to more and more weaknesses.

Peacemakers tend to learn a great deal about a few things and become expert in those areas, the guru. President Carter studied to be an engineer in the nuclear submarine program at the U.S. Naval Academy (Annapolis) and maintained an avid interest in advanced sciences throughout his life. After his father's death, he contemplated leaving the Navy, going home to farm, a decision he never thought he would face. True to his personality flaws, he chose to face the dilemma alone and did not involve Rosalyn. Besides being uninvolved, he admitted he became self-righteous, discouraging and indecisive. The silence was very stressful. He felt disloyal to the embryonic nuclear submarine program; they had saved NO money to enable them to up and quit and go home (they had watched it!); and they could not expect to make money by farming because peanuts were selling for only one cent a pound. Carter knew nothing about farming his Dad's peanut farm or any other commercial enterprise. Gross proceeds from working an acre of peanuts would yield seven dollars an acre. For that $7, he would buy or save seed, break the land, cultivate it at least seven times, plow up and shake dirt from the peanuts, put them on stacks, let them dry, thresh them and haul them to market, and find enough money left to support his family. Could he find his true **Millionaire Code** learning to be a farmer? Questionable.

When he made up his mind to go home to farm, his behavior sounded more and more like the stubborn weaknesses of a Peacemaker. As he put it in his autobiography, Rosalyn — who was the opposite of her spouse's personality — "rebelled in every possible way, ...resentment was bitter and persistent...we made the long trip (from New York to Plains, Georgia) in almost complete silence." He took quiet, justifiable control in silence; after all, the Peacemaker thinks that *one person* has to *quietly* take charge and manage resources, time, friends, work locations, and work assignments.

Taking control of self is good; taking total control of others is not good. It leads to resistance, challenge and face-to-face *"internecine warfare."* And this is exactly what happened. President Carter admitted that he faced doubt and fear of failure, but he did not want anyone to know he was vulnerable. Unfortunately, failure was a possibility.

They moved into a tiny apartment with three young sons (Amy was just a glitter in their eyes) in a public housing project in Plains, Georgia, in 1953. The first year, he struggled with the farm supply business, made much worse by one of the worse droughts in history. After investing all their savings and what he could borrow in an inventory of seed, fertilizer and other supplies, they finished 1954 with a total income of less than $300 and a mountain of debt. Their $10,000 loan application was rejected, but they were able to secure a small line of credit from a customer and netted a profit of almost $3,000 the following year (for the whole year). Ups and downs in the farm business may build character, but it certainly didn't build capital.

His expressed leadership in his Baptist Church combined with running for office in his small town started him on the right path to live in strengths. He soon entered politics, fought for civil rights and over the next 20 years served as a Georgia State Legislator, Governor of the "Empire State of the South," and then President of the United States. Throughout his political career he was forced to face additional weaknesses, doubt and failures. Learning the hard way, however, his communication improved: In "the political world, where we all faced common challenges together, our family has learned to resolve difficult interpersonal issues by communicating." We're sure this saved Rosalyn's sanity! The Peacemaker's silence can be deafening.

When he left the Presidency, he once again *"faced bankruptcy as well as the self-doubt, private losses, and disappointments."* During his Presidency, the Carters left the warehouse business in the hands of financial trustees. Upon returning home, they found themselves almost a million dollars in debt (a lot of debt in the 1980s)! The farm business was in shambles. Luckily, an agricultural corporation decided to enter the peanut market, buy their warehouse, and pay them almost enough to pay off the debts. Together, they made a good decision, sell. Once again they were free to pursue core strengths and, as they say, the rest is history!

To sum up, Peacemakers are inherently great listeners and money watchers! But they are not extroverted, great speakers, or even good communicators *until* they learn and lean toward their strengths. Carter's leaning toward weaknesses in his Peacemaker DNA (dollars, numbers and attitude) preceded his financial night-mares. Watching his money idle or handing it off to professional outsiders made for risky business. On the other hand, in his later years, still armed with his peacemaking **Millionaire Code**, strengths served him well — strengths such as persistent and thorough attention to dollars, numbers, attitude, generously sharing time and money, communicating with opposite personalities, attending to details and assuring that money goes where intended.

Peacemaker Personality #2
Clark Howard, The Master Of Saving Slow And Steady
(A.K.A. Cheapskate — and we mean that in a "loving complimentary way.")

Clark Howard is the multimillionaire radio host on WSB-AM in Atlanta, Georgia. Nationally syndicated, he opens his daily show with the following statement: *"This is your daily consumer-empowerment zone. Our goal? To help you pack a punch in your wallet and find better ways for you to save more, spend less and avoid getting rrrrripped off."* He uses his strengths to delight of his audience and the stations that carry his enormously popular program.

What are his Peacemaker personality strengths? He is a tight-wad, a *silhouette* with* a "golly-gee-willikers" everyman persona, inoffensive and pleasant with callers. He has that dry Peacemaker

---

*What is a silhouette? Etienne de Silhouette was a deficit-fighting finance minister of France in 1759 who had the nerve to suggest raising taxes. The nerve! To this date his name is synonymous with cheapness (*Reader's Digest*, Dec 2001).

humor, perfect for the slow, steady pace typically needed for solving financial problems in consumer life.

For five hours a day (unless he is testing his own travel advice), he sits or leans on desks in his stocking feet while he educates listeners to be gurus in wealth accumulation and preservation. He is known to deliver cheapskate advice in pithy, parsimonious Benjamin Franklin-like proverbs. When someone is making a financial faux pas, he cues up the siren for the money police; or if they are about to get ripped off or scammed, he releases a barking pit bull on the sleazy merchant. He is a focused listener and mediator par excellence, a Peacemaker stepping between consumer and merchant when he perceives mistreatment. He strongly values fairness and seeks balance between consumers and businessmen. Like all Peacemakers, he values self-reliance, patience, and a saving lifestyle.

Clark Howard's upbringing was the opposite of President Carter's. He was the youngest of four children in a very affluent family. He lived in a posh Atlanta neighborhood and attended the finest private schools and summer camps. His family's affluence was owed to his grandfather, the "bra mogul" of the Lovable Company. He lived a life of privilege and comfort. So how did he become the "cheapskate guru?" He came home from college one Thanksgiving to learn that his father had been fired from his job. "There was barely enough to pay for the rest of the school year. After that, I'd be on my own". How could his parents have so much money and with one setback end up with nothing? Howard describes their financial personality as one of conspicuous consumption, a *"grasshopper approach to finances."* They debited out by hopping from one expenditure to the next.

Howard left college and went to work full-time as a civilian employee of the Air Force. He attended school at night graduating with a degree in urban government three years later. Having learned by necessity to be money conscious, he pursued a master's degree in business while working full time for IBM (which offered full tuition reimbursement, the start of good deals). He invested part of a $17,000 trust fund started by his grandfather in an electric-car company that promptly went belly up. He calls this second experience with financial loss "sobering." Not one to miss a third strike and be out of the game, Howard put the rest of the trust fund in stocks and set out to get financially educated.

He studied the business news and learned about airline deregulation. He invested the profits from stock investments in a chain of travel agencies. He told *Kiplinger's* that "I sensed there was a growing opportunity anytime an industry opened itself up to competition. Thank goodness, I was right; that industry just went bonkers." The travel agency business led him to opportunities in real estate, and he invested additional time and money in rental properties. Six years later, Howard sold the chain of travel agencies to an investor group for $300,000. That sum and a frugal lifestyle, plus rental income sheltering tax savings allowed him to retire at the age of 31.

Although retirement didn't suit him, his frugal lifestyle did. Even today, a multi-millionaire in his fourth decade of life, he buys his clothes at an inexpensive department store, and everyday purchases (even eyeglasses) from a warehouse club. In keeping with Peacemaker profiles, he hates malls. He buys pre-owned cars, store brands, used furniture ($99 for a sofa) and everyday purchases from warehouse clubs. When he shops, he refuses to take a shopping cart. As he put it, "I walk around with stuff in my arms. Eventually, it gets heavy, cutting the shopping trip short."

His cheapskate philosophy even relates to travel. Direct airplane flights are overrated, he claims. Being inherently *adaptable and obliging* (there's that Peacemaker DNA!), he believes time is overvalued if saving it squanders money. He has been photographed waiting in line to get the cheapest gas in town. But his overriding message is not to figure out how to cut corners, but to save the money **before** you have to cut corners. He stashes 15% of pretax income for retirement and 25% of after-tax income for readily accessible (and peace of mind) savings. He turned to systematic investing because he figured he knew only enough to be dangerous with stocks and bonds.

In *USAA Magazine* (May/June 2002*)*, he said that systematic investing takes the emotion out of withdrawing money for savings. He admitted that his index funds and mutual funds are valued much lower per share during a down economy, but looking at it from a longer-term perspective (like he does), the potential for gain is greater. Continually adding shares monthly at sale prices means "for the shares I'm buying now, I'm getting much more bang for my buck."

In addition to socking away money for retirement and for both sunny and rainy days, he simply spends less than he makes. And we only wish we made what he saves because he makes a lot! Howard's annual salary is purported to exceed $1 million (remember, he's still in retirement). He airs on 150 stations, is featured on TV and writes periodic columns in the newspaper. He flourishes in three homes in three states, all "tastefully decorated" (*Kiplinger's* observations, not ours) with warehouse and used furniture. He and his wife, an actress, relax in his backyard pool, game room and media center. He is not against spending if you can afford it. "People try and put me in a bargain box. That's not my deal. I'm not into deprivation. My philosophy is defer, not deny." pg. 112).

Obviously, he does not deny his family. In fact, he sounds like the peaceful mediator at home. He can afford to be. He buys discounted personal goods for himself but bought his wife a substantive diamond at, of course, a warehouse discount store. He forgoes shopping with his 12-year-old daughter because she does not share her Dad's zeal for frugality. Howard admits "We have a don't ask, don't tell, don't pursue policy," which may be interpreted to mean that he will (on occasion?) throw money at situations to keep the peace.

So, what can we learn from Clark Howard? Being conscious about strengths, dollars, numbers, and attitude precedes being and acting really rich! For example, financial advisors tell us to follow our instincts, a key to future behavior for any personality, but those instincts may not always be financially sound. President Carter's decision to go home to farm when he knew nothing about farming may have been right personally, but it was not good for financial wealth. At that time, he was not fully conscious of peacekeeping strengths. Howard's instinct to get into the electric car business was financially disastrous. When he wasn't clear what his inherent strengths were, he tried investing in new fad industries and stocks on the advice of family and peers. When he recognized his strengths and his weaknesses, he applied the principle of systematic investing in stock and index funds and will never be in a *"financial worry zone"* again.

Instincts are trustworthy *if* we know our DNA or dollars, numbers and attitude strengths, and are willing to get educated before we invest. Consciousness should precede action. If we don't recognize what is good for us, we are likely to take advice that may only work for someone else. We often ignore what seems obvious and easier to us because everybody is doing and recommending something different. But, what comes "easy" may reflect inherent personality traits, those qualities that are individual to you. Remember, what is easy for one personality is difficult for 75% of the population (e.g., the other three personalities). What is inherently easy for the Peacemaker may not be intuitive, easy or even desirable for the Problem Solver or the extroverted Pleasure Seeker or Powerbroker. Get educated! Use your inherent strengths and lean away from flaws.

Peacemaker Traps

As a rule, Peacemakers do not avidly pursue money, but they want and need it for financial status and clear conscious. And that's ok. But flip it around, does limited financial status mean no status and no peace of mind? Peace of mind is akin to self-worth that comes with confidence in decision-making, conscious behaviors within each person's **Millionaire Code**. Obviously, limited financial status doesn't equal limited self-worth. If self-worth and peace of mind erroneously equal top-flight financial status, Peacemakers are more apt to lean toward weaknesses (e.g., depriving themselves, denying family money, exerting a quiet will of iron or stashing money away, even "under mattresses"). They often forget there is another option.

First, if you're a Peacemaker, lean toward inherent strengths.

What do you know best? What are you most interested in? What are you willing to do and learn? How do those answers relate to and make money? Second, define what specifically contributes to "financial status" and "peace of mind." Be realistic, list the reasonable elements such as source of income, readily visible savings for a specific time frame, comfortable housing, reliable transportation and insurance. Specifically define what "secure" personally means, without the constraints of being perfectly secure. Educate yourself (with and without help), devise a plan, accumulate and preserve money methodically, slow and easy. Once you have "financial status," you must monitor it for safekeeping but develop a plan that allows you to responsibly "chill out" from deprivation. Avoid leaning toward weaknesses that may let doubt, worry and fear of the unknown, fear of not understanding money, dominate behavior and never really build wealth.

A related financial trap for Peacemakers is that they do not like change. If they anticipate problems (which they hate) and have to make substantive changes, they can become fearful and subsequently worried about money. The resulting behavior is to remain hesitant, even aimless procrastinators. If they are also non-communicative, the financial problem often escalates both in corporate offices and boardrooms as well as at home with family. Should the problem get bigger, deteriorate, and come down to no money (e.g., foreclosure, bankruptcy), this personality loses status and all self-confidence. Unlike Clark Howard or President Carter, they often lose the instinct to land on their feet. It takes a lot to change thinking and affect behavior like these stalwarts did.

A third trap is being aimless about savings and investments. The reasons are many. Either (1) they are not educated (remember, if they can't be a guru, they hand off the job); or (2) they are not inclined to develop a financial plan (remember, e-a-s-y, not hard); or (3) they are *easily* diverted from the plan for a "cause" (mediating others' problems). All three problems have solutions but the third is the most difficult in which to compromise. Although it is *admirable* to lend support to family and friends in need, Peacemakers are known to satisfy a perceived crisis first and very slowly or never return to their financial plan. Accumulating financial wealth naturally involves attaining and balancing tensions between individual and others' needs.

Peacemaking Strengths

The Peacemaker is compassionate and concerned about individuals, which is good. They are excellent listeners, observant and make excellent people managers, encouraging others to think for themselves and to land on their own two feet. They prefer to keep the peace and avoid confrontation, letting other people shine. As long as earnings are good and loss statements few, the Peacemaker can start early with a steady financial wealth building plan, pick a safe avenue for designated savings and enjoy compounded interest. The biggest strength for this peaceful personality is patience.

Exercise your strengths: Competence, patience and perseverance. Get educated about money, start early with a regular saving and investment program, and plan for change instead of responding to crises, thereby avoiding interruptions. Make automatic deduction transfers to investment plans that will escalate with compounded earnings. Check in with family and business needs often so as to avoid crises, which spell trouble, new and unwelcome responsibilities. Even gurus can and should ask for help in order to reach the balanced lifestyle they desire.

Millionaire Code Stories

For Love Of Family Or Love Of Money

Joanne and Gene have a lot in common, especially a wonderful sixth sense about generating and successfully amassing a lot of money. While very wealthy, their financial personalities, specifically how they see money and how they spend it, do not reflect shared traits. The recession years made that very clear.

Joanne is a Pleasure Seeker with money, and Gene has a Peacemaker **Millionaire Code**. Gene is more and more entrenched in weaknesses since retiring (for the third time) and seeing the darkness of a three-year recession through his age 60+ eyes. Joanne does not understand her repeat conversations with the wealthy

Peacemaker. All he ever seems to say is "We don't have money for that," "We have to go on a budget," "We're losing everything," and "We can't afford that (trip, dinner out, clothes, etc)!" She loves to travel abroad; and when anyone is available, she also enjoys trekking off to their mountain cabin, their beach house, or the old family homestead. All properties have ongoing expenses, however, as well as value. Gene is threatening to sell it all while Joanne, being an optimistic Pleasure Seeker, continues to live for today and trusts that tomorrow will be better.

Gene, on the other hand, has become one with his reclining chair, the financial news station on TV and harbors a semi-permanent negative pout. Typical Peacemaker flaws are readily visible: He dampens enthusiasm for anything, stays uninvolved and indifferent to plans, judges other's spendthrift ways, resists change, is very hard to get moving, discourages others, lacks self-motivation. Regardless of how fearful and worried he is about his sinking savings and retirement plans, he falls prey to the Peacemaker weakness of doling out money to keep the peace. Joanne is watching while he helps grown, working sons pay for their health, auto insurance and, of course, their charge card bills.

The latest hardship that required Gene's money was for a first cousin that was worried about keeping their business during the financial slump. Sensitive, caring and doomed to help, Gene responded with a loan. However, what is a loan between family? It is an ambiguous cross between a donation and an expectation that the loaner would be repaid "someday." One gave, and the other received. There was no paperwork, no interest discussed, and no agreement about repayment terms. The business fortunately turned around in six months, but the cousin then succumbed to his spouses' wish for a new house. The borrower did not offer to pay Gene back first. Moreover, what's a new, big house without nice, brand-new furnishings? This family furnished their house with lavish surroundings and invited extended family in for a reunion to celebrate their success. They did not offer to pay Gene back first, second, or third. To date, there's appears to be no intention to pay any borrowed monies back. The Peacemaker regrets, frets and fumes, but will not ask because that would present a problem! Problems require a close look at responsibility, so it's easier to just feel guilty.

Consciousness precedes change in behavior and action. Gene and Joanne thought they never had different approaches with money. After all, they were quite successful with wealth attainment. But Gene thought Joanne was the only big spender between them, at least until they took the financial personality test! But, he was a big spender, just in a completely different way. They are still in disbelief now at how opposite they are in financial spending behaviors. Gene understands that his behavior around money is showing, and it frustrates Joanne. His behavior says, 'I want you to be just like me,' (fearful and worried, unenthusiastic, resist change in these times of uncertainty, and just sit down and be with poor me). Too bad! He's married to a Pleasure Seeker, and she is just not going to do that because they can't change their optimistic DNA. He did not plan on that!

He envies her strengths; but he still thinks he'll just watch while she remains cheerful, emotional and demonstrative in tough times, and energetically living in the present. He is re-evaluating the secure plan he made for retirement in order to get realistic, instead of melodramatic, about the limits the current economy poses. He promises to make necessary changes to increase peace of mind and reduce existing high risks (those stocks that were supposed to come right back after their crash). Peace be with them — or at least with one of them!

Velvet and iron hands

Born during the depression, and a textbook "Rosey the Riveter" during World War II — she was the chief cockpit engineer on the B-29 — Deenie B. is a 77-year-old Southern doyenne with the textbook iron hand in the velvet glove. As you might expect, she's a textbook Peacemaker. Introverted (as a result, Deenie B. is not her real name), she wants to keep the peace no matter what. However, if she ever has to take a stand, she will, and look out for iron-clad quiet will of iron! She's an example of someone who did not need to risk principal, AND one who saw that her strengths were intricately tied to her weaknesses (notably one who resists change from certificate of deposits and resents being pushed to bonds by bankers who refuse to pay her a fair interest).

She has no faith in the stock market, and that's final. She has never been victimized by any get-rich scheme. However, in her mind, there's only one way to get money — the old fashioned way, to earn it. Over the course of her long life, she's had good luck with consistent and boring safe certificates of deposit. Even now she will tell you, "There's probably other places where I could make more money, but I'm not going to lose my principal." And that has been her watchword all these years, "Save but don't lose your principal. You may need it some rainy day."

Recently, she's found herself in a difficult situation. She came to the authors with a problem and a request generated as a result of the bear market of 2002: CDs are coming due and "Make me safe." As she put it, "The banks ought to be embarrassed over the low rates. Who do they think can live on that kind of money." Nevertheless, she's lived too long to "lose my money now."

What to do? She took our money personality test, zeroed in on her DNA financial weaknesses, and turned them into strengths. She was not going to give in just to make peace with bankers. She did not fall prey to fear and worry, indecisiveness or self-righteous behaviors typical of Peacemakers leaning toward weaknesses, resisting change, being indifferent to all suggestions and plans.

She was willing to learn how to research bank rates and U.S. savings rates until she found just the right place to put her money (for her personality, her age, health and stage in life). She did not go home that afternoon and stuff her assets "under the mattress" (e.g., the "affectionate" term financial advisors use to describe CDs and money markets earning 2-3% interest), and she did not procrastinate until she no longer felt despondent. She asked herself the right questions at the right time, used her administrative abilities, remained good under pressure and found the easy way for peace of mind.

As she put it, "Where can I find a safe haven for my money — one where I can get to it when I need it — one where I can watch it steadily grow, and still make more than the banks are willing to give me." Watching an old 1940s movie on Turner Classics, the film ended with a plea, the film actress reminding, "War Bonds can be bought in the lobby of this theatre." There it was! There was her answer. Re-harkening the days of World War II — quite a patriotic young, old woman — she followed through and checked out current U.S. Savings Bonds. She found they were offering a better rate of return than these "'selfish' bankers." She found the answer.

She located an "I" bond that was paying the same rate as the banks plus an extra bonus. The bond she settled on paid a guaranteed rate of return, plus a changeable rate of inflation — total rate almost 5% at publication. If inflation went up, so did the interest payment; if down, well, she could trade it in with just three months penalty. She sat down, did the seventh-grade math, and realized that even if she had to trade it in, she would make more — even with a penalty —

than the bank was offering.

Moral of the story in her own words: "I may not be the best with money, and now I know where I'm weak. I will take my fear of losing money and let it motivate me to make as much as I can and still feel like I've protected my principal." Had she invested in something riskier, her own peace would have been jeopardized, and she would not have been able to live with herself. Smart girl. For her it was a smart money choice, and it is her money. Now, she laughs, "I thumb my nose and walk by all the bank VPs who tried to scare me into a 2% certificate of deposit. I found a higher rate, and a safer one. I'm not going to pay for their big houses or their sports cars!"

CHAPTER SEVEN

The Pleasure Seeker: Let's Do It The Fun Way!

7
∞

Financial Pleasure Seekers are popular people magnets. They value money for love and fun. Money is a way to expressively entertain self, family and others in fun ways, parties, vacations, sports, and activities of all kinds. The little girls knew how to charm dads, and the boys knew how to appreciate moms. As children, they typically started out as "the popular kids." They talked early and constantly, convincing peers and teachers that they had the "best personalities" and were someone others should follow because they do fun things. As adults, they use their financial **Millionaire Code** in professions that emphasize flexible hours over schedules, glamour over work, creativity over routines and people over statistics.

Pleasure Seakers are inherently compelled to talk to anyone about anything. This is a strength they use to teach, act, lecture, buy and sell in any venue. They can find the newest and best purchases that enthusiastically please others. They want and need to be appreciated for locating great buys that sincerely express happiness and enthusism for life. They are shoppers par excellence and are very good at planning and finding that all-purpose purchase (e.g., novelty groceries, houses, clothing, cars, boats, and vacation get-a-ways). If they choose to focus on creatively investing in real estate, stocks, savings plans in the same way they focus on other purchases, they can easily use their strengths to join the 3.5 Club. Investments can be like shopping. Thank goodness for good, old-fashioned fun. So, how do the pleasure-seeking professionals unlock their **Millionaire Code**? How does this work in the real world? Check out the following examples of Pleasure Seakers in the popular press.

The Many Faces Of The Pleasure Seeker

Personality #1:

"BODACIOUS" MARY FOLEY: Age 33, Retired and Independently Wealthy

Mary started at AOL (America On Line) at age 23 as a customer service representative making $8 an hour. She had an engineering degree from Virginia Tech but had already decided not to use it, much to her parents' dismay. Pleasure Seekers hate deadlines and details. As a result, she must have intuitively known that an engineering career was not a particularly good fit for inherent personality likes and dislikes. She followed her **Millionaire Code** (instead of her degree) and chose to work in the people-oriented communications field. Interestingly, she says that accepting the job at AOL was "… dumb luck, navigated only by my intuition" (a favorite word for expressing personality).

In her book, *BODACIOUS* published in 2001, Foley says she "loved the adrenaline-charged environment where so much creativity, vision and innovation were harnessed." She was promoted and managed corporate training for the next decade. To retire wealthy at the end of that period, she must not have spent like typical Pleasure Seekers. She had to have saved, invested in corporate stocks and 401K plans that performed exceedingly well throughout the 90's.

Somewhere in the initial years of the AOL-Time Warner merger, the pace quickened, demanding a high degree of organization in order to meet training deadlines. Organization takes a lot of routine work, scheduling, statistics, the opposite of glamorous, creative, or people oriented. The fun was coming to an end.

She was burning out. Stress often shows up as physical first, and she noted that she was losing sleep and easily distracted. You know you need to make some changes when you forget your dress clothes for work! She actually had to go to meetings in her exercise leggings one morning because she forgot her pants. One particular training rollout had been all consuming, and AOL-Time Warner recognized the job no longer fit the person. She lost a promotion opportunity (to a man hired from outside the company) and when she lost her fun, lovely, private office with a view of the lake, she knew something had to change.

And something did change. She adopted her **Millionaire Code** and embodied it in a battle cry, *"Bodacious"*, which she defined as "vigorous feelings of being courageous, creative, larger than life, self respecting, being completely, madly, thoroughly, full-speed-ahead, exactly who you are and relishing the experience, with apologies to no one." Whew! She retired from AOL a wealthy woman but her life was just beginning. She started her own company, "Bodacious" where she is a success coach, inspirational speaker, and author. What does Mary say now about unlocking her financial abilities, her **Millionaire Code**? "I'm not afraid anymore of my own confidence...I'm not afraid anymore of letting my vulnerabilities show, ...of showing my power, experience and expertise...."

In *BODACIOUS*, her "rules" for success — abstracted and paraphrased here — are rules that Pleasure Seekers can live by:

1. **Talk to Yourself.** People pleasers tend to talk to everyone else and forget to look within until they are forced to after some negative event. When this personality is feeling stressed and anxious about flaws and weaknesses, their inner voice tends to come down hard on core behaviors, punishing mistakes. Mary tells us that our *true* inner voice is *supportive, simple, honest* and best of all, *gentle*.

2. **Respect Yourself.** Review which strengths come naturally and which do not — plan to use what comes naturally and learn the rest.

3. **Surrender to Change.** Improve the quality of your inner message, e.g., how you speak to yourself, be more prospective instead of punishing.

4. **Show Off Your New Behaviors.** Experiment with more confident behaviors congruent with personality, showing your compassion, verbally communicating, reaffirming that you are listening.

More likely than not, those changes show up in your checking account.

Pleasure Seeker Personality # 2

Tim Sanders, Chief Solutions Officer, Yahoo!

"Nice, smart people succeed (NSPS)." That is Tim Sanders' primary message to audiences and admirers who come to his seminars to learn how "NSPS" can work for them. In his book, *Love Is The Killer App*, friends and coworkers describe him as creative, articulate, fresh, energized, inspiring, enthusiastic, and provocative — in other words, all the trait strengths for a Pleasure Seeker. His motto is "Love — not speed, technology, shrewdness, or meanness — is the killer app(lication)," a phrase used in the personal computer revolution of the 70's and 80's. It does appear that his behavior and personality are congruent with his millionaire financial code.

Tim's star was definitely on the rise in the 1990s as Yahoo was the preferred search engine on the internet for millions of users. Advertising dollars were flowing in, and he excelled as the corporate "lovecat." What is a lovecat? "I believe that the most important new trend in business is the downfall of barracudas, sharks and piranhas, and the ascendancy of nice, smart people. He was evangelizing, sharing and growing, "...realizing the fruits of my lovecat ways." But his strengths were intricately tied to his personality flaws, and in his book, he admitted he crossed the line.

He blew it. Tim fell prey to typical personality flaws. He related in his book that he missed big opportunities for his personal and company's financial growth when he got so energized that he *"had a gazillion balls in the air."* He did disappearing acts with potential clients and blundered under the demanding time and organization stresses — potential traps for this personality. He missed emails and phone calls, forgot to follow up with people. People had come to expect the "lovecat" follow up. "There was just too much buffering going on inside my head — I didn't have enough personal bandwidth available." Slowly but surely, clients disappeared and re-appeared making big money for other people. After that short diversion from his **Millionaire Code**, he returned to his "lovecat" ways.

Tim's "rules" for success, paraphrased from *Love is the Killer*

App and re-written below, adhere to the Pleasure Seeker **Millionaire Code** of behavior:

1. **Understand Limits.** As the lovecat system begins to kick into gear, be careful not to overextend yourself, to overestimate what you can deliver.

2. **Be Prepared to Be Burned.** Showing compassion is an inherent strength but can leave you feeling vulnerable and, if rejected, hurt. Before taking rejection personally, think again about what the other person needs. Seek to create win-win situations and solutions with others.

3. **Have a Backup Plan.** Have a plan, and then have a back-up plan in case that one fails. It'll give you the extra confidence to get it done. If at first you fail, then do it again, right!

4. **Read Above Your Grade Level.** Read in depth about subjects you need to know, especially the ones that may not be fun to digest.

Pleasure Seeker Traps

The Pleasure Seeker is on the exciting, fun track. They are "now oriented," preferring to live in the endless instant. The present holds the most promise. For this personality, the future may never get here. In fact, they believe that one can *never* live in the future. This line of thinking has been a downfall for many.

If they don't pay attention to stresses and weaknesses, money flows through their hands like water. One minute, they can finish paying bills and enthusiastically commit to pay off all charge cards. The next minute, they'll use the charge card "just one more time." When they succumb to their weaknesses, they lose sight of the truth and do not have the funds to finance more fun. Pleasure Seekers are easily tempted to spend anything from greenbacks or plastic to IOUs and promises. They can agree to a financial plan but buy stocks on margin or bid on a designer item, promising to pay by charge card. This personality has great difficulty with the small details. They are big picture thinkers, and often forget to pay the light bill.

Pleasure Seekers Strengths: Satisfy Wants And Needs

Pleasure Seekers are excellent shoppers who can stay on task and ferret out good purchases and great investments, if they choose to focus instead of throwing money away. Whether the stock market or the real estate market is of interest, they can use inherent strengths by talking to experienced, knowledgeable people. Building a network, a team of working professionals to pull together the tax details, wills, portfolios, real estate, insurance (homeowner, health, car, disability, etc), is a highly valued step in wealth creation, for Pleasure Seekers in particular. They can easily find out what criteria is important to understand about investing in company stocks, as well as what they need to know about shopping for location in the real estate market. Visualizing and pulling together the big financial picture comes easy.

Asking for help with the details, accounting practices, and feedback on plans for tomorrow is a necessity! Do not take the "fun tract," and borrow to invest, combine insurance with investments, or pawn off tasks you don't like on other professionals. The outcome of not knowing what you are doing is an open invitation to fret and worry. Try looking specifically for, interviewing, and working with opposite personalities. Perfect Problem Solvers, for instance, love to tract the details you don't inherently know how to use but need. Spend less than you earn and pay off any high-interest credit cards. Finally, in order to preserve lots of extra cash flow for shopping, do invest and use an organizer. Missing bill-payment deadlines, overlapping credit limits on multiple cards, not tracking charges and debits can eventually ruin love and fun.

Millionaire Code Stories

Oh, For The Pleasures of The Single Good Life

Brian is a very successful clothes salesman. Handsome, debonair, he looks great up front and is very passionate about colors, fabrics and cut of shirts, coats. The big picture all has to come together for him and his lucky clients — lucky that is if they can afford custom suits at $4,000+ a clip and all the dress shirts with French cuffs! Many, many people can, do, and should if they have their wealth sewed up, so to speak.

Being a 29 year-old Pleasure Seeker with money, he thought he was in heaven during those last five years of the 1990s boom time. He inspired people to join his list of elite customers and charmed them to recommend him to their friends. He loves people, makes friends easily — what a great people job, going from audience to audience and making them laugh and be happy. Plus, he had his own enviable closet of custom suits and shirts, only the best shoes, a personal trainer every morning at 5:30, a sports car and absolutely no thoughts of leaving the bachelor world at age 29. That was "yesterday."

This is "today." Post stock market highs, Enron, WorldCom, Global Crossing, Andersen, and all the companies affected by those scandals, the CEOs, CFOs, accountants and lawyers are not ordering new custom threads. Matter of fact, annual sales fell 10% in 2001 and more again in 2002. Gentlemen are examining the half-price sales of the finest suits in the retail shops. The newest trend, however, is to buy personally made to measure suits between $800 and $1300 at retail. Brian never saw what was going to hit him; after all, he was not part of the high flyers in the "dot.bomb" business busts, right? How could clients go back to retail? Easy! But how could he return to low commissions and high expenses with virtually no savings. Hard! While he still has a way to go to pull out of his personally created financial trappings, he has rallied.

He developed his own battle cry and sees (some) humor in how typical he was as he plummeted into his personality weaknesses. Loving the work, he decided to work with his company to develop a line of stock patterns like the retailers were using in made-to-measure suits. Working with his personal trainer's clients and their referrals, he enjoys working with the man who lifts weights at the gym and can't get his big shoulders into a suit that fits the rest of him properly. Will he put away money for tomorrow this time? Absolutely! Will he resolve his expensive problem for the leased sports car? Certainly! He even has one steady girlfriend. Lucky for him, his personality strengths are intact, ready to be of service when he leans toward them.

The Problem Solver:
The Right Way Is The Only Way!

8

Every circle of friends must include the perfectionist Problem Solver. They have an almost magic, inherent ability for understanding the importance of details. Misusing a word, a period, or a comma in the wrong place drives them nuts. Not only do they appreciate finer products (quality more than quantity), they prefer to buy the "best" of a few things until they can have the "best of everything." In casual conversation, they're easy to spot. To explain, when asked, "How are you?" they typically answer, "Fine." What they're really saying is "Things aren't perfect, but this is as good as things get, and that is just *fine* for now." Given this approach, they are cautious spenders, analyzing and researching each detail. To that end, they express their money skill when it comes to detailing budgets and taking the necessary time to analyze the best values for lowest prices. They prefer to follow *the right way* to *the right plan* and NEVER compromise on the details. However, too much of anything is no good.

The Problem Solver, like every other human being, occasionally falls prey to weaknesses. Chasing the dream of perfection can cause them to tire of trying to right every wrong. For example, more than any other personality, they value a neat house, office, and desk but are often the messiest housekeeper. Why? They know whatever they start, they expect to finish perfectly. They get bogged down in the details. Being perfect and doing things right is often just too hard!

When things do not appear right, they are easily depressed and either reluctant to do anything or dangerously impulsive. When the right solution at the right time does not happen perfectly right, they can turn fiercely independent and resort to the extreme of doing nothing or demonstrating an impulsively flippant side. When they see the errors of their ways, they are very, very sorry — full of guilt and remorse.

How does this guilt play out with money spent on purchases? They return more than they keep, of course! After all, they meticulously made lists of what they wanted, researched every detail, and started shopping for the purchase months ahead of time in order to find the perfect item. The Problem Solver may have even collected coupons, studied newspaper advertisements and examined records of purchases for the same category in the past. They organized their shopping, refused to get side tracked by a clown or a "special" in the store and only bought when the purchase was deemed a good investment.

When they make the wrong purchase, buyer's remorse kicks in. They realize they're stuck, but they have the ability to learn from their mistakes. They vow never to make the same error twice, freely teach others about their stupidity, and in many cases, seek revenge against the evil doer who sold them the product. Their revenge is always legal and typically in the realm of "I'll tell others about you," and "I'll never shop with you again." In other words, they try to get back at those who hurt them through the pocketbook — where they think it will hurt them the most.

Overall, their winning strengths are a matter of balance, staying true to their money credo without becoming overly obsessive-compulsive. Somehow they tend to stay detail-oriented, economical-minded, analytical, orderly, and organized, all at the same time — they can be truly mental money jugglers. Being conscientious, they are logical and schedule-oriented. They might begin planning for retirement early in their careers, picking slow and steady investment strategies for the long haul — and scoff at asking for help because they *should* be able to learn what they need to do. This personality doesn't think they need professional financial assistance until they make their first million. However, unless they are professional financial analysts, they rarely have the time and inclination to "perfect" their investing knowledge and skills. Just like "perfect" housekeeping is often postponed, "perfect" financial plans materialize late, if ever. See how this personality faces strengths and weaknesses in the real world.

Problem Solver Personality #1:

Natalie Cole: Multi Millionaire – Problem Solving Vocal Artist with *An Angel on Her Shoulder*

In Natalie Cole's autobiography, *Angel on My Shoulder: An Autobiography* (2000), she portrays herself as a woman struggling to be "the best." She desires to be perfect in all ways, as a daughter, spouse, singer and performer. Born into the world of glittering privilege, she is the daughter of legendary singer Nat King Cole, one of Hollywood's most famous families. As she explains in her autobiography, she has known severe poverty, having been homeless and addicted to heroin on the streets of Manhattan. Like every human functioning in today's real world, her strengths were tied to her weaknesses. Problem Solvers seek to be purposeful and serious, creative, idealistic but can flip into being full of contradictions, disliking opposition, and have a deep need for approval. She instinctively recognized this when she wrote about one particular trait, *"impulsiveness."*

Natalie described herself as impulsive, as having a propensity or natural tendency to step out on a limb, grow and pursue a singing career despite her mom's disapproval. It enhanced the adventurousness in the Problem Solver that, for her, enabled her to try every kind of musical style. However, she felt it fueled many mistakes, and even Webster's dictionary notes that impulsive behavior is not always rational. "Impulsiveness has also been my curse. It has made me foolish."

She let her impulsiveness lead her away from performing the kind of music that came easily and naturally to her. When she was 23 years old, she obstinately chose Rhythm and Blues (R&B) music. Typically, young Problem Solvers are inherently unhappy unless everybody likes what they are doing. Not everyone liked her R&B music, and she was not happy! Rather than pursuing her strengths in music, she ran away from them, saying she "was not gonna sing 'Nature Boy' to a bunch of living fossils in leisure suits just because they'd been stuck in a time warp for 20 years. They were snobbish and clueless, and I was stubborn and on the defensive."

Three different times, Natalie denied her strengths — her artistic and musical talent, her drive for perfectionism, and high standards. She fell prey to her flip-side weaknesses — being fragile, insecure, and extremely introspective. Expressing that melancholy, deep need for approval, she was sure everyone only paid her attention because they knew her father. She never felt as though she knew who her friends were. Burdened by living in her father's shadow and insecure that she could *never* be as perfect as he, she set out to be her opposite, a people pleasing Pleasure Seeker. However, she was who she was. She wanted things to be perfect, to be accepted by the "confident, happy white kids." That respect would come much later, only when she realized that she had her strengths and individuality.

In keeping with her idea that only people pleasing extroverts succeed, she did whatever it took to be "popular" and to fit in. Acceptance and popularity were paramount. When her boyfriend shot heroin, she had to try it. Soon, addicted to heroin, she recounted episodes of homelessness on the streets of Manhattan. When a fellow addict showed her how to print up bogus checks — she had to try that too. Nothing was too high or too low.

When did she finally know what was good for her? In the late 1980s, she returned to her roots. She recorded "Everlasting" in 1987 with Burt Baccarat using her perfectionist millionaire DNA. Her real comeback, however, came in 1991 with the multi-platinum album, "Unforgettable…With Love" a tribute to her deceased dad. Using her genius prone DNA, she dubbed her voice over his and created a duet; but success was only tentatively tied to strengths.

Weaknesses got the best of her, and her life careened out of balance again. Just as the album was being awarded seven Grammies, her marriage collapsed. Laden with emotional and financial issues concerning the divorce, drugs, deaths of loved ones and even her mother's lawsuit, she "had all the self esteem of a squashed grape." It wasn't until she recorded "Stardust" in 1997 and her "Greatest Hits" in 2000, that she forever returned to her strengths found in her millionaire financial DNA. She reported feeling strong and comfortable with her personal style. Introspection and reflection are important to the perfect Problem Solver who is inherently a sensitive and faithful personality. Hope and gratefulness, not to mention a strong faith in God, sum up her story.

What's the lesson here? A Problem Solver who tries to masquerade in pleasure seeking clothing will fail until they become true to personality leanings. It is one thing to value and try to learn from opposite personalities and something else entirely different to mask up as a different person. When Natalie's behavior reached congruence with her inherent personality, then she enjoyed the success she so wanted and deserved. Can someone coach or beg her to make changes? Not easily! Can she change herself, her behavior? Of course! By knowing inherent strengths and weaknesses, she can decide to be open to experience and not be jealous or threatened by the riches of others.

How many times have you taken advice on attaining success or riches from someone whom you admired? If you are like us, many times you've tried to perfect what works for someone else. What looks like a winning formula fails because we underestimate the unique differences in personality. Know and lean toward personal strengths, away from weaknesses, and enjoy the success.

Problem Solver Personality #2:

J.B. Fuqua, Consummate Entrepreneur With "OPM"

J. B. Fuqua is quite the inspiring rags-to-riches story. Advocating the intellectual manipulation of "Other People's Money (OPM)" to amass extraordinary wealth, consummate entrepreneur, the perfect Problem Solver and accredited genius, bought or sold over 40 companies, from radio and TV stations to bakeries, trucks and lawnmowers. At age 80, he shows few signs of slowing down in his autobiography, (*J. B. Fuqua: A Memoir*).

As a youngster, there was no money for a college education so he borrowed books from the Duke University business school and educated himself. He was a sponge for details, numbers, and accounting methodologies that fit his millionaire DNA. And consistent with others who share this financial personality, he's also known for being helpful and unselfish with others. True to form he later rewarded Duke's generosity with his version of largesse in the form of building the Fuqua School of Business. However, that was far from the end of unselfish sharing of fortunes. He's contributed millions of dollars to promote awareness and reduce the stigma of severe mental illness. Almost a modern-day "Frasier," he is sophisticated in art, music, literature, thoroughly enjoying the details, funding multiple performing arts centers for youth.

Apparently J.B. is a "perfectionist" in everything including his appearance and business deals. Like a lot of introverted personalities, he prefers to surround himself with small groups of close friends and working cohorts. Typical of this personality, they prefer deep conversations with a few people, again quality over quantity. He likely tolerates parties, but probably does not love them. In fact, Problem Solvers tend to dislike parties where stories or jokes are bantered about which can insult and hurt feelings. His sensitivity and sense of right and wrong in the community led him to passionately serve in the Georgia State Legislature.

Again in keeping with his financial **Millionaire Code**, he is very precise in what he says, thinking before he speaks so he doesn't say the wrong thing. He wants all the facts before making a decision so he can do a thorough job. He is very reliable and keeps a tight schedule so he knows what to do next.

So, did he ever have any weaknesses? He was said to be workaholic, a behavior that is known to sap personal and family energy. Granted, workaholic behaviors are not limited to perfectionists; after all, any of the four personalities can take strengths to excess and lean toward weaknesses. However, unable to rest, perfectionist workaholics typically experience periodic explosions of pent-up anger or residue of negative feelings. They tend to find fault, get down in the dumps, moody, even nervous. He admitted he has "lots of ego," but he certainly needed that to borrow and to invest billions of other people's money in the buying and selling of 40 companies. Ego was good, but again, strengths are intricately tied to weaknesses and are a matter of balance.

What he didn't need, but grappled with for 20 years, was extremely poor health. Poor health can change the landscape for wealth management. Admitting to workaholic weaknesses off and on throughout his autobiography, sleep was rarely restful, and he was often fatigued. He withdrew from close friends and family and found himself in the throws of a severe depression. After 20 years of successful leadership, there was a serious miscommunication with his Board of Directors. Fuqua described the opposition and subsequent break in relationships as devastating and antagonistic. When thrown into chaotic situations, Problem Solvers dislike those in opposition because they typically block their goal. The goal and the introvert's strength is to find creative solutions to problems, but being too introspective blocks open communication with different personalities. There was the expected period of stagnation and dullness, with the subsequent loss of accountability. The company was ultimately sold.

Does the story have a happy ending? Interestingly, the purchaser was Fuqua's opposite, a controlling Powerbroker leaning toward his own weaknesses. He attempted to drastically change the personality of the company and fairly quickly went bankrupt. He explained, "Watching a company I had built up over more than 2 decades be destroyed in such a (negative) manner was devastating to me and took years off my life." J.B. saw it coming; he bought back his name for $1 million and secured his reputation. What did Fuqua conclude about the real Problem Solver's millionaire DNA?

We studied his analysis and have abstracted his billionaire rules for Problem Solvers below.

1. **Details, Details, Details.** If you don't pay attention to the details, then work will be rewarded with re-work. A little time and planning initially pay big dividends later. Being *organized* and making sure the *right* thing happens at the *right time* requires time and planning.

2. **Find the Advantage**. Here, Fuqua emphasized honing your ability to communicate a message as well as paying attention to how you deliver that message. This personality is credited with concrete and precise language. A Socratic approach to problem solving, however, can be a put off to other personalities. Statistically, one-half of the population visualizes the big picture while Problem Solvers and Peacemakers focus on detailed issues as a means to finding the advantage. Among the big picture takers, half want the fun way, and half want the fast way. The Peacemakers want the easy, peaceful way. Beware, the problem solving *right way* for you may not be in others' vernacular. Concrete, judgmental thinking about what other's say or worse, what you think they say, is a prime example of leaning toward weaknesses.

3. **Quality Preferred**. J.B. chose to invest in promoting color TV, which he considered "quality." Conventional wisdom at the time dictated that quantity was the way to go — stay with the "tried and true" black and white. The latter was where the millions were at the time. Color was the future. He took the right step at the right time and obviously, this decision contributed millions to the industry. When J.B. says pay attention for what "looks like a good deal," he expects you to ensure that your research and education back the idea. Quality over quantity.

4. **Strike Now; Delays Cost Bucks**. *If* you are educated and your clearest vision, highest thought is to act, don't give into perfectionist skepticism, pessimism, and the need to squash disorder. These are trait weaknesses for the perfect Problem Solver. For example, "One of the ways that fortunes have been made is by buying real estate on an interest-only basis." If you don't have cash for your clearest vision, investigate alternative out-of-the-box thinking and methods of financing. Interest only loans, balloon payments at strategic points when you project success and using other peoples' money are legitimate ways to act now.

5. **Make Conventional Wisdom Unconventional.** Fuqua said, "If I had paid attention to conventional wisdom, I would not have accomplished one tenth of the things I did." For instance, going forward with the production of color versus black & white TVs was against conventional wisdom. He knew very well that hidden in conventional wisdom was a logic that could turn a new-fangled unconventional idea or product into a conventional one.

What's the lesson? All perfect work and no spontaneous play rarely work for any personality. While the Problem Solver tries, he cannot be all things to all people and tends to put himself in 2nd place to his work. That's never smart, even if you have billions to keep you warm on cold, cloudy, emotionally empty winter nights. Functioning at work is adjunctive to other personal needs, family, friends, finances, fitness, and faith. There is spiritual wisdom in balancing wants and needs.

Problem Solver Traps

The perfect Problem Solvers are typically skilled at many activities that use the detailed thinking processes. These thinkers are just as likely to pursue millions through art, music or writing as they are to orchestrate highly skilled businesses, computers or even rock climbing and safari adventures. Their source of power comes from their ability to assimilate details, in serene calmness and silence. However, in times of conflict, this calm silence can lead them to withdraw, delay, or avoid risk completely, suppress personal emotions and generally be inaccessible, generally confused and messy with their **Millionaire Code**.

When they get close to financial success, their primary weakness can be a rise in self-doubt, subsequent need to squash disorder, and a retreat to whatever looks like security at the time. Natalie Cole doubted she could succeed unless she changed herself from perfect Problem Solver to popular Pleasure Seeker. She saw security in what the popular group did and to break away would introduce disorder and insecurity. J.B. Fuqua orchestrated order and disorder *perfectly* until he fell prey to being the extremely perfect entrepreneur with forty irons in the fire, addicting himself to workaholism. What Fuqua didn't know — but found out the hard way — is that workaholism additionally produces neurochemical changes that can and do affect health status. All work, no rest, withdrawing from family, persistently demanding the perfect decision right now, the resulting exhaustion and depression lay heavy burdens on the spirit of personality.

A secondary weakness is that Problem Solvers have difficulty balancing the need for order over disorder. When leaning toward strengths, they are critical, nit-picking analyzers of purchases and investments. When leaning toward weaknesses, they are critical, nit-picking buyers. So, strengths equal weaknesses, how do you know the difference? They may assess each purchase or investment with a critical eye and make an educated decision. On the flip side, they will slow to a stop with a negative attitude, doubt, and insecurity because they *expect perfection, an illusory concept.* If they wait for perfection, they won't choose any path. Withdrawing and eliminating all chaos with finances can lead to procrastination when opportunities vanish. Inherent weaknesses can easily rule over strengths. Finances dominated by doubt will never build wealth. Security versus freedom is a choice.

In an effort to be economical, orderly, security conscious, a third weakness for this personality is ignoring the need for a tax plan. As a result, they tend to pay excessive taxes and interest payments. Robert Kiyosaki (more on him later) noted that the security conscious person pays the steepest price later in life, right when retirement plans are ready to kick in. All 401K plans, Series E bonds, stock and other bond liquidations have tax ramifications and each is different. An educated, detailed approach to addressing the need for security can keep this personality out of financial traps.

Problem Solver Strengths: Satisfy Wants & Needs

Perfectionists do not like uncertainty, disorder, and especially chaos, not in classrooms or boardrooms, personal expenses or corporate finances. This affinity can work to their benefit if they lean toward their strengths, away from security traps. Rest assured that billionaire financial plans pay attention to details. Accept and appreciate strengths and satisfy the perfectionist skepticism.

Problem Solvers must have security. Don't allow this to be an amorphous concept. Define security! Satisfy this need by designating how much money needs to be in accessible emergency savings (for example, three to six months of earnings) and make it a priority to secure this amount in an insured money market, certificate of deposit (CD) or savings account. In his book, *The Wealthy Barber*, David Chilton methodically coaches how to shore up property and other current investments with the security of health, property, disability and liability insurance. Determine an amount to cover expected down payments on immediate investments, homes, cars, vacations, unforeseen expenses, and repairs. Develop a tax efficient risk plan to face health concerns or career changes with peace of mind. This satisfies "security."

Build in a point for *educated* risk taking. After all, this personality is associated with genius DNA, so get educated about all three things: dollars, numbers and the right attitude for you! Along with the security of following a financial plan for wealth building can be the freedom to reexamine dreams. Be aware that life has its ups and downs, and don't toss out freedom when they bring some disorder, some chaos. Perfectionists have to balance the tension between perfect order and total chaos if their nascent creativity and wealth building strengths are to be utilized.

What is it like for a Problem Solver who has just spent too much money?

One perfectionist client bemoans, "I hate money. I hate what it does to me, and I hate what it does to other people. But most of all, I hate the pressures which come with it, or more accurately, the pressures which come when you're short of it." Typical of so many creative types, Kenny B., goes on: "And who can be productive and imaginative when they're having to deal with bills, investments, and other daily money pressures." So, what does he do? When the money's tight, "I go into shut down mode. I don't spend nothing [sic] on anything. Instead, I go on a tear; I call everyone with whom I do business and give them a money ultimatum." Here's what he means. "When the money is tight, I call everyone who bills me on a regular basis and get them to lower their prices." What's really interesting about that, is that nine out of ten people he calls will lower their bills. He explains his technique.

"First I called the security alarm people, I advised that I'd never had a false alarm, that I had been with them for 5 years, and that I wanted a price break." They said, "Okay." The result for Kenny B., a reduction in costs from $24 to $18 a month. And it doesn't stop there, when Kenny B. starts on his money hit list, he's like a gangster with demands. "Then I called my credit card company and demanded a lower interest rate and free service. They complied. Once again, I explained, I've been with you for years, never had an overdue bill, and if you want to keep me, then what are you going to do?" According to Kenny, they gave him a "sweet deal — lower interest rate and no yearly fee." He goes on, "And then I called the TV cable people and shut it down. Besides, I need to be reading more, and TV time was dictating my life, and lowering my IQ. And finally, the phone company. Just didn't need all those fancy bells and whistles they talked me into. Cancel 'em."

So, how does he deal with tough times? When he's forced to deal with money, he turns from a mild-mannered Problem Solver into a mega-watt Powerbroker. Anyone who comes in his path is subject to his saying, "I want a lower price." And while he typically would just pay and go, when he reaches his weakest limit, he rebels, reacts, and puts his money life back on track. So far his total monthly savings from this one angry outburst is around $300 a month. All this pro-active stuff has put control back in his corner, and now he can be creative again.

"No" doesn't always mean "no"

Problem Solvers are sensitive and have high standards. As a result, they tend to interpret communication from their own personal perspective and often forget that what you say may be different from what they think you say. To explain, Problem Solvers are very precise with their words, and they think everyone else is that precise. Absolutely untrue! For example, there are at least four different ways of interpreting the simple word, "no." People laughed when former President Clinton said, "It depends on what your meaning of 'is' is." One of our seminar participants learned this the hard way.

Kevin is a certified financial planner and textbook Problem Solver who had trouble with the fact that the simple straightforward word "no" has four different meanings, not one. As a Problem Solver, Kevin thought "No" meant "No, I'm not interested." That's exactly what it means if one Problem Solver is meeting or working with another Problem Solver. But for Problem Solvers and Peacemakers, it could mean, "No, not without all the details, charts and 5 year earnings tables!"

If a Pleasure Seeker and Powerbroker say, "No," they could mean, "No, what's the point? I don't see how that fits in the big picture."

After completing **The Millionaire Code** 16-question profile, Kevin got an education and an epiphany. Being the sensitive Problem Solver with money, he took "No" to mean that the client was negative about his suggestion. But no means more. If you're an introverted personality (Problem Solver or Peacemaker) "no" means first give me access to money details and time to analyze. If you're an extroverted personality (Powerbroker and Pleasure Seeker), a "No" means, "I need the big picture first before we can even think about a 'yes.'"

The Powerbroker: My Way!

9
∞

The Powerbroker has *real goals* for building financial wealth, and money is the means by which they finance their productive vision. The goal may be mastering specific educational-related tenants, starting a business, or buying a big-ticket item. As natural goal setters, they have the uncommon ability to follow through.

Whatever it is, the Powerbroker has the ability to search out the best deal on products or services. As a result, a pat on the back, an appreciation for their goals, action-oriented plans, decisiveness, and success at running anything is appropriate. Simply put, they are exceptional in their ability to aggressively tackle, finish a job (no matter how distasteful), and implement a plan to grow riches fast.

Another of their under-appreciated, yet incredibly sharp abilities is their very, very practical shopping acumen. Almost as if they keep a mental map of perceived needs — for themselves and others — they rarely choose a playful or fun gift without having first been told someone wanted it. Most gifts are useful and for a specifically observed need. For example, one of the authors is a Powerbroker who gave the love of her life a warm-up suit for a cold, wintry "Happy Valentine's Day!" The romantic, pleasure-seeking partner didn't much like the gift. But that's just the way Powerbrokers are. They are practical even when they shouldn't be — even in romance. Because they have confidently organized and planned each and every event (including romantic holidays), they prefer to control money and all shopping experiences. In grocery stores, look out for them. Their cart is a bumper car — speeding around aisles, in and out as quickly as they can! It's curtains for the salesperson who tries to pull the wool over their eyes. Powerbrokers have been known to reduce salespeople to tears. When shopping for clothes or other items, they move at a fast clip, are like a magnet to their exact purchase, and woe be he who gets in their way.

Also, don't ask them to stop too often on a road trip. Avoid excess liquids, and better take a picnic basket full of snacks. They are a personality on the fast track! At intersections, the driver in front needs to be ready to spring forward when the lights change or get an impatient honk and a verbal, "Move it." Powerbrokers like to drive, and that is good news for opposite personalities, who prefer to read, daydream or watch the scenery. They prefer and want to be in control. The bad news: In the midst of traffic and frustrations, the Powerbroker is likely to drive around in circles, fussing and fuming, and never stop and ask for directions. Problems are challenges that raise their passion levels.

Their credo is simple: "See a problem, fix it fast, and do it economically." Quite willing to tackle a challenge, they find an answer, get the job done, and move on. The solution needs to be fast and sure, *and* accurate, too. The easy or fun way is not an option (that would take too much precious time to ascertain). Do not get in their way. They do not suffer fools easily.

Each and every day begins with a mental checklist of what needs to be accomplished to make it a *good* day. They want and need to check items off an invisible list prior to addressing any personal, family or cohorts' add on to-do lists. Some Powerbrokers are so compulsive they prefer a written "To Do" list to a mental one. These people methodically check and re-check. In fact, if they do something that was not on their list, they write it down — even hours after the event — for the sheer pleasure of crossing it off the list. Their "To Do/Done" list is a mark of achievement. While many of them are moving toward the electronic palm pilots, a true Powerbroker is quite content with his written list (some are even attached to the dashboard in their car). An electronic device just can't duplicate the pleasure of crossing an item off the list. "Delete" just doesn't feel as good. They need to see what they crossed through as a sort of mental reference.

They are change-oriented, perhaps even driven to create change. Their goals pay homage to the future; that is, the future as far as they can see. They tend to have less patience with long-term plans, retirement savings, or buy-and-hold (and hold and hold) investments.

Finally, the Powerbroker thrives on competition and is easily bored when cooperation is required. Their competitive spirit is a critically important strength for wealth building; however, it can get in their way. For instance, cooperation is needed with long-term savings, investments and relationships. Too often, we see the Powerbroker giving "it" all they've got and losing it because their competitive "gotta change it now" mentality got in the way. If only they could have cooperated just a bit more.

In the real world, here's how Powerbrokers play their strengths against their weaknesses.

Powerbroker Personality #1:

Alex Spanos, Sports Aficionado

Alex Spanos is the owner of the San Diego Chargers, purchased in 1984. As a noted philanthropist, he holds the "Statue of Liberty-Ellis Island Medal of Honor" and the "Horatio Alger Award." Like other Powerbrokers, he instinctively set goals for himself. In his autobiography, *Sharing the Wealth*, this Greek billionaire credits his "dreams" for his goals and success. Rush Limbaugh, the famous radio talk-show host noted in the introduction that "no" simply isn't in Spanos' vocabulary; "negative thoughts never enter his mind."

Spanos earned his first million by age 33 in 1956, five years after he quit the security of his family's business. Working at the family's Greek restaurant and bakery until 1951, he learned a great deal about service and money, but still felt he "could do nothing right." In *Sharing the Wealth*, Spanos related, "My three brothers followed the family plan. My brother, George, became a lawyer and could do no wrong in my father's eyes."

Though Spanos did not clarify, we guessed that his brothers

were opposite personalities from him, ones who were like Dad and personally thrived in the close-knit family structure of the Greek restaurant business. Unlike them, he wanted and needed more power, self control and took off on his own, borrowed $800 to buy a truck and started his own catering business. Credited with being an entrepreneurial "genius," he excelled in the business and quickly expanded and diversified into real estate and construction. Alex had limited formal education, only his dreams, but appeared to have a heads up on his personality code.

Not all of his dreams could be realized so quickly. By age 50, his net worth was one billion, so he added another goal: To build another billion in the next 10 years. He bought the Chargers in 1984 and set the goal to be Super Bowl contenders by 1987. Setting personal goals worked great. Setting goals for teams of people put him face to face with the myriad of Powerbroker personality weaknesses. To accomplish his goal, he appeared to fall prey to Powerbroker thinking that the end justifies the means. He demanded, dominated, bossed, and had little tolerance for mistakes. Five years passed before he enjoyed one winning season with eight wins and seven losses. Those wins were followed by more losses, not exactly Super Bowl material, yet! Five more years passed and his goals were eroding on his fields of dreams. "I truly believed in my heart that we could build up the team and make it to the Super Bowl in five years. But I was wrong."

The reality was that his failure was ironically due to his strengths, but strengths taken to extremes become weaknesses. He was an adventurous, persuasive, strong-willed, competitive, resourceful, bold, daring, confident, and decisive Powerbroker — all admirable financial personality DNA. But examine the downside of the Powerbroker personality.

During those ten long years he was described in the book as "impatient," "argumentative," " a workaholic," "domineering," "tactless," "intolerant," "headstrong," "stubborn," and "short tempered." Pressures reached a feverish pace. His health eroded and a heart bypass followed. Spanos recalled the losing years from 1987, "Losing was a new and terrifying experience for me. Some

Monday mornings, I'd shut the door to my office at the Chargers' headquarter and actually cry. Other times, rage would overcome me."

The coaches called him a "live volcano." But behind the blustering facade, he recalled that he was suffering, becoming clinically depressed. The team lost for eight more, agonizingly long years. If that was not enough, the fans verbally booed him during the 1988 loss to the 49ers.

In the end, he reevaluated his strengths, being tenacious, independent and positive thinking — all the traits we value about Powerbrokers. Spanos related that he recognized which negative strengths were getting in the way. *His* personal involvement and *his* hard work mattered little to the *team's* win-loss record. By enlisting the *cooperation* of the players and management, he helped to figure out what the Chargers wanted and needed. He recognized he could lead and still let someone else manage. He was ready to cooperate with other personalities and back off to win. Winning the 1995 Super Bowl was the ultimate reward for cooperation and creative teamwork. Once he relinquished control over others, reestablished self-control, he was able to sit back and enjoy the fun aspects of owning a winning team (and rake in the financial gains).

In summary, Spanos recounted that "success has three key elements: vision, desire and instinct." Paraphrasing from his auto-biography, *vision* is knowing what you want (e.g., the dream). The *desire* propels, provides momentum to see the vision accomplished. *Instinct* (another of our favorite words for personality traits and personal spirit) serves as a compass for making the right decisions at the right time. Spanos' experience illustrates how essential it is to return to basic *instinctive strengths,* your personal **Millionaire Code.** Our vision of the lesson learned is that competition without cooperation makes for a blustery financial and emotional experiment.

Powerbroker Personality #2:

Robert T. Kiyosaki, author, entrepreneur

Robert Kiyosaki is a fourth-generation American of Japanese descent, born and raised in Hawaii. A millionaire by his early 30s,

Kiyosaki did not retire until age 47. Why? In between times, he hit his personality weakness head on. In his first book, *Rich Dad, Poor Dad,* he recounted that his retirement was the result of rediscovering his strengths and getting educated. He sought out a personal trainer, enthusiastically, passionately, much like a boxer before a match. He was the only student and his "trainer" was a billionaire — his "rich dad."

Kiyosaki graduated from college in New York, joined the Marines, and went to Vietnam as an officer and helicopter pilot. Returning from war at twenty-something, Robert went to work for the Xerox Corporation and saved $3,000 to invest with his best friend and his friend's rich dad (thus the name of his first book, *"Rich Dad, Poor Dad"*). But they turned his money down. Why? His $3,000 savings were not enough to "invest" with the big boys. That amount of money was only sufficient for rainy day savings, something Powerbrokers don't particularly value. Young Kiyosaki had his first lesson about business in the real world, assets and liabilities, income and expenses, and investment technicalities. He experienced the 90/10 rule first hand.

The 90/10 rule summarizes the wealth paradigm. His friend's rich dad observed that 10% of the people have 90% of the money. The average person is in 90% bracket holding only 10% of the monies. Kiyosaki simply refused to be "average." The average investor seeks total security. People who seek only security often miss out on freedom. His biological father (the *"Poor Dad"* in his book) valued security. The elder Kiyosaki advocated making good grades, finding a steady job with a strong future and a pension, putting a few dollars aside, and accepting a reduced income for a secure retirement 50 years in the future. Young Kiyosaki rejected his poor dad's **Millionaire Code**.

Determined not to follow in his father's footsteps, he left Xerox in 1978. He admitted he was nearly paralyzed with fear as he resigned and collected his last paycheck. Striking out on one's own typically involves risk. Risk involves mistakes. Mistakes can be costly. Could he stomach risk? He started a company that brought the first nylon Velcro surfer wallets to market. The company made millions and then lost those millions. Why? He thought all the different personalities who worked with him were just like him, wanted the same things he wanted, and valued money the same way he valued it — for freedom, independence, not security or peace of mind. Kiyosaki soared using his strengths — productivity, creativity, self-reliance and confidence. He crashed by being headstrong, impatient, and resistant to learning the cooperative ropes in business from the flip side or flaws in his personality.

> "The way to great financial wealth is to strengthen your strengths and address your character flaws. And the way to do that is by first recognizing them rather than pretending you are flawless." Kiyosaki, *Cashflow Quadrant: Rich Dad's Guide to Financial Freedom.*

Kiyosaki's experience and insight has made him an expert in predicting financial behavior. This insightful, humbling quote acknowledges that personality strengths and flaws affect the accumulation as well as the losses of money. Understanding how your personality drives money away or pulls it to you is the first step in joining the 3.5 Club as a sustaining member. With this realization, it's possible for each of us to be sustaining members. Once we understand the personality mechanism that motivates our family members and co-workers, we can check off their strengths on our mental checklists. Then it's possible to make educated guesses about how these people who are so important to us see and value money. When wants and needs for each of the four personalities are identified, it's much easier to take the steps necessary for altering weaknesses that prevent our millionaire DNA from spinning off the financial spreadsheets.

Young Kiyosaki did just that. He acknowledged the problem that after his first business experience, he had no money, zip, *nada*. He and his young wife were homeless and gratefully slept in a friend's garage. He had to start over and create financial assets without the ability to buy those assets. Rich Dad challenged him to fill a blank asset diagram with financial assets, no purchases allowed. His "job" was to "create assets" where there were none.

This job and challenge was very different from his Poor Dad's job and life lesson. Well educated but financially average, Kiyosaki's father was an educator, ultimately vying for the position of Superintendent of Education in Hawaii. He had a good job that paid well and would provide permanent job security. Poor Dad expressed what many Problem Solvers believe, "I believe I'm secure, why do I need to invest?" In reality, Poor Dad was locked into a high-risk mindset and totally trusted someone else with his money and his future freedom, in this case the government and the Teacher's Union. He was not educated in the ways of business and investing and was content to trust that his savings were safe. The problem is that the job world and job security paradigms change, and they do this often. The elder Kiyosaki lost his job when the politics no longer valued his moral stance. By the time he was able to see that his pseudo-safe environment provided no security, he was unable to digest the impact and rally. Instead of meeting his expectations of being financially secure and even free in his final years, he was dependent and destitute.

Kiyosaki observed Poor Dad's financial typhoon in its total cycle, from enjoying comfortable, secure finances when he was eight, to financial turmoil and high stress in his teens to financial ruin and dejection by young adulthood. Over the same time period, he observed his best friend's Rich Dad become visibly richer and stress free over time, investing and creating more assets along valuable Hawaiian beachfront properties. Surely, no one person could afford all that, but Rich Dad said his business could. He created assets and now was home free.

So how did Young Kiyosaki choose to create assets and freedom? He became a business owner then an investor. He investigated franchises and "business systems." He was not afraid to take on good debt — borrowing to purchase an investment that has *proven* to grow in value. He avoided taking on bad debt — borrowing to buy lifestyle purchases, a fancy car or stocks that can and do go down in value. He described one real estate investment where he bought a large property with a house on it, sold part of the land and the house, and used the money from the sale to invest in building his home on a portion of the vacant property. With careful research, planning and execution, the former sale easily paid for the latter and the entire transaction was an asset. From this initial investment he developed a "system," created a real estate company and invested in apartments and then office buildings. Each time he gained tax advantages and reinvested gains. Currently retired, he's still spinning gold from authoring books, seminars and investments.

His Powerbroker "system" included building a network of successful friends, entrepreneurs, investors, and the people that make businesses hum (for instance, certified financial planners, lawyers, accountants, tax professionals, estate planners, real estate and stock market professionals). He resisted and never "controlled" them; he just controlled himself. His goal was to work hard for portfolio and passive income. Portfolio income is generally derived from paper assets such as stocks, bonds, and mutual funds. Passive income is generally derived from real estate or income derived from royalties from books, patents, or license agreements. Passive income from real estate has three benefits, (1) rising property valuations, (2) monthly rental income and (3) substantive tax advantages. Passive income is a highly desirable commodity because it multiplies whether you are asleep or awake, at home or on vacation. He set out to get rich; he made money to save; and he saved to invest, not to spend (not at first anyway).

He diversified further by investing some profits in direct distribution systems. For example, he realized that for $200 he could join an existing network marketing system and immediately start building a business. Due to technological advances in computers, these network-marketing companies are totally automated. The headaches of paperwork, order processing, stocking, distribution, accounting and follow-up are almost entirely managed by *the business system*. New distributors focus all of their effort on building a business instead of worrying about the normal start-up headaches of a small business. These business systems offer incredible business education opportunities from hands on mentors as well as providing the education and support on how to lead people. He believed, like so many wealthy people have discovered the hard way, that making $1 million is sometimes the easy part, keeping it is tough.

What's so hard about staying in the 3.5 Club, about making and investing larger and larger sums of money? Inherent strengths are tied to inherent weaknesses. When things are going good, we rarely review, diversify and make changes. But as Kiyosaki learned, we need to keep learning and innovate, innovate, innovate. His Rich Dad always laughed at the investors who kept pushing their wheelbarrows around in circles thinking that the investments and dividends would always be there each time they come around for them.

What's the lesson? Opportunities for achieving wealth and freedom are multiple. Optimism and the competitive spirit are welcomed strengths. But Kiyosaki specifically observed how important it was to acknowledge and pay attention to weaknesses, specifically those related to controlling emotions with money.

The Powerbroker Trap

To build wealth, the powerful personality struggles to manage the inherent and nascent tensions between competition and cooperation. As Donald Trump explained in *The Art of the Deal*, "Money was never a big motivation for me, except as a way to keep score. The real excitement is playing the game." Many Powerbrokers can lose track of the small moves that shore up "winnings" along the game board because they are excited about the big picture winnings. They end up going for the score and get mad when the score is zero. Unfortunately, as "The Donald" found out, it's a double-edged sword. Competition (to win) and cowardice (to cooperate) can fuel their weaknesses and behavior.

The Powerbroker can easily get caught up in winning for its own sake, losing sight of the need and value of cooperation. They can discourage disagreement and are firm in their persuasiveness of a strategy on the fast track. However, their inherent need to win can overshadow any need to ensure that others win, too. Their thinking is that if you're nice, you're not tough. The choice becomes their way or no way. "I win, you lose" is tough, yes, but courageous? No. It is cowardly.

The cost of overusing competition is expensive: destroyed relationships, loss of cooperation, anger, depression and stagnation of wealth. On the other hand, history provides ample examples of societies devaluing competition in favor of cooperation. It is no different for the Powerbroker working in a family or cooperating in a business. In tandem, competition and cooperation create valuable riches.

Powerbroker Strengths: Satisfy Your Wants & Needs

The Powerbroker is the most sought after speaker on the lecture circuit and, based on our observational research, the most prolific autobiographer in the bookstores. They set goals and dive into projects with vim and vigor and tell all. They really get things done. While this personality represents 25% of the population, it characterizes nearly 75% of the authors and CEOs writing and lecturing on the "rules" for success. What's interesting about this picture? The other three personalities make up 75% of the audience who are trying to read about their opposite's **Millionaire Codes**! Remember what Kiyosaki learned — one personality does not always have the right answer for someone with different wants, needs and values, i.e., alternative DNA.

Powerbroker success strategies work best for *naturally* goal-oriented personalities. The benefits of their approach are speed, decisiveness, and preservation of their values. The weaknesses of their approach include speed, decisiveness and preservation of personal competitive values *when* further reflection and common sense says otherwise. Not everyone can successfully implement the Powerbroker's fast pace and mental map of success. Demanding or controlling the pace for others won't make things happen, no matter what! Powerful **Millionaire Code** propel them to take charge of themselves and the situation, which is good, but their strengths become weaknesses when they take full charge of others. There is a difference between leading and creating a forced march. Other personalities may not be able to implement their charge, stopping cooperation in its tracks, which then comes across as insubordination to the Powerbroker.

Cooperating with pleasure seeking, problem solving and peacemaking goals is often "the 'X' that marks the spot." Understanding how the four groups build on each other is where the wealth lies. Experiences related by both Spanos and Kiyosaki are a testament to what happens when they blustered through uncooperative poor choices to go it alone. When these billionaires repented, did an about face, reevaluated right and left brain assets, and decided to cooperate instead of just compete and dominate, they were able to refocus their compass and make lots of money. They have millions (loving family, friends, too) and contribute to communities. The point is that the Powerbroker can benefit from other "team" members at work, at home, and in the community

---

AVERAGE DEBT IN AMERICA

The average individual credit card debt = $2,411.

Holding the average amount on three different cards will amount to $7,233 in principal. If your cards charge 18% annually, you are paying $1,300 for the stress of borrowing for things you cannot afford. Sometimes charge cards can run up to 21% APR. Check your truth in lending disclosures. If you are a good credit risk and on a mission to pay off debt, ask for a lower interest rate!

Millionaire Code Stories

The DNA Powerbroker Credit Trap

Carmen and her husband are two career professionals, a highly successful couple making six-figure incomes, but they could not keep from maxing out charge balances on credit cards. "My husband and I considered ourselves ahead of the game, you know, 'financially well-educated.' And we were, there's no doubt about it. We pulled our credit reports every six months, religiously doubled our monthly payments on credit card balances and STILL couldn't figure out how we owed over fifty thousand dollars to various credit card companies." Carmen took the money personality test and after counseling with the author, she became conscious of playing to her and to her husband's weaknesses. She was a Powerbroker (big spender), and he was a Problem Solver (big saver). She wanted to find the fast way to live right, and he wanted to find the right way to live securely. Time was of the essence for two busy professionals and charging goods and products originally reduced stress. In a deadlock between a spender and saver, they got lazy with finances and adopted the Peacemaker Money Operating System (MOS): if it's not broken, don't fix it. However, they were not conscious of their strengths, and their actions were not congruent with potential membership in the 3.5 Club. Their MOS was broken. Charging lifestyle and debiting out every month became its own stress instead of being an answer to stress. In order to wean them back into living within their means and lean toward their strengths, they were instructed to pay themselves first! Here is how it worked for Carmen:

We figured out that the few credit cards I had that were paid off were the one's I NEVER used. I didn't want to charge anything on a card that had no balance. We closed those immediately. The second thing we decided to do was start paying the minimum due every month. I balked at this in the beginning until one of the authors explained that we were going to take the overpayment I always paid and put it in our money market. You see, our personalities were such that we could never get out of debt because even though we were making astronomical payments, we could still not see the light at the end of the tunnel. The author recognized this and had us stockpile the extra money until we had enough to pay the entire card off. To date, we have only three of the five $10,000.00 card balances left and haven't created any new debt.

The Gift List For Wishful Partners

GIFT LISTS FOR FUN, POWER, SECURITY, PEACE OF MIND

PLEASURE SEEKER'S Fun Gift Wish List:	POWERBROKER'S "Take Control" Gift Wish List:
• Planned events/tickets/lessons around favorite *social* sports like tennis, golf, bowling, dance. • Love high-tech conversational gadgets that don't require detailed expertise but keep them talking, communicating, in touch, socializing. • Active "fun" vacations, mountains adventure. • Freedom to be creative and entertaining, e.g., photography, cooking, gardening, golf/art/craft/dance/acting classes. • Time to talk… with family, lots of friends. • Celebrations, talking and sharing stories. To have fun with happy people. • To be appreciated for humor and engaging conversational ability. • Happy upbeat music, cards by snail/email. • Sunny sunflowers, professional or hand delivered in front of an audience • Lucky colors: yellow, orange. • Jewelry is good for both genders. • Parties! Parties! More Parties!	• Sports aficionados; Tickets or lessons for *powerful, control-oriented* sports; e.g., all Olympic sports, football, tennis, golf, weight lifting, fencing. • They want you to passion-ately support their fast track for a goal. • Promise to help with their *to do list*! • Organize their closets, schedules, phone/address lists, calendars for them. • To always have something to do, to look forward to, e.g., a special event, trip, new car. Future goals are fine. • To be appreciated when they take charge and direct projects (…of course, where someone else will volunteer to handle the details). • Self-improvement vacations, books, tools, seminars; fast, fastest computer software. • Intricate high tech gadgets, watches, stock picking and financial planning aids. • Lucky Colors: Passionate red, clear black • Flower: red, red roses

PROBLEM SOLVER'S Perfectly Detailed Wish List:	PEACEMAKERS Easy Track Wish List:
• Art and music aficionados, e.g., books, ticket to concerts, museum trip, photography or art/dance/cooking lessons (maybe in France/Italy?) • To be trusted with details (checking, savings) and given the time to finish. • Vacations that use talents for precision: Snow skiing, ice-skating, parachuting (really!) • Quiet time for reflection with lots of books, magazines, herbal teas (fresh flowers, candles) • Value shopping for short periods of time (very budget minded); plan your purchases/trips specific to personal interests, "little things". • Loves special bows, wrappings, lots of special attention • Compassionate novels and ballads. • Surprise, sensitive, thoughtful email cards/calls, flowers: bluebells, pansy. • Lucky colors are blue and purple • Beta fish, water ponds • Beaches!	• Comfortable, lazy furniture; peaceful decor. • Love nonfiction books in history, philosophy, nature, coin/stamp collecting. • Books or new gadgets related to topics within their "guru" expertise or hobby • Time relaxing alone, or with a *few* close friends, e.g., hunting, fishing or beach trips; no tight schedules. • Vacation from "to do" lists • Financial security, stocks, savings, low debt • Help with shopping; Prefer shopping at small, mom and pop shops • People watching @ Starbucks, movies • Low key vacations or sports like walking, golf, all spectator sports. • Lucky colors: white, green; flower: daisy • Beta fish inside and fish or water ponds out • Peaceful music, classical CDs • Green grass and a great mower

CHAPTER TEN

How Opposites Attract & How To Make That Work

10

∞

Opposite personalities have different pet terms for "MONEY". Take a look at these thesaurus terms according to *Roget's 21st Century Thesaurus* correlated with financial personalities. Which of these fit you or your spouse best?

- *Pleasure Seeker's* "creative, fun" approach fits the following synonyms: wealth, opulence, affluence, riches, fortune; *Slang,* fast or quick buck, ways and means, wherewithal, almighty dollar.
- *Problem Solver's* practical "right" approach with money meets these synonyms: finances, funds, treasure, capital, assets, competency, solvency.
- *Peacemakers* save a lot so their accessible greenbacks are meager and make life easy: petty cash, pocket spending, mad or pin money, change, small coin.
- *Powerbrokers* save very little but think big and fast for adequate control: rich man, capitalist, financier, millionaire, multimillionaire, billionaire; rich as Croesus, Midas, tycoon, heiress. *Slang*, moneybags, zillionaire.

There are a few certainties in life: Opposites attract, and partners fight; and they fight over finances more than any other joint issue. Whether you want to learn more about your individual scores or maybe you're one personality and your mate is another, either way, the following chapter will answer the question: How do we relate to each other when it comes to money matters?

Most people have a primary and secondary personality. Some people are strongly compatible with one **Millionaire Code**, and others are equally divided between two codes. Littauer warns in her book, *After Every Wedding Comes a Marriage*, that some personality combinations are healthy contrasts; others are not *naturally* compatible and make thought processes more challenging. For instance, an individual may be a Problem Solver with money at work and a Pleasure Seeker with money at home. Each of the personalities value money differently — they do have opposite **Millionaire Codes** of behavior. It is highly likely that one of the conflicting personalities is inherently and naturally you, and you learned the second approach from influential others. Learning different approaches to money is good; otherwise, how else will we learn to do unto others as *they* want.

However, if for years, you have been trying to satisfy someone else's demands and expectations about how you make and manage money — and it is not working — you may lose more than you gain. You need to be true to yourself. It is time to reevaluate your strengths. We are looking to capitalize on your natural tendency to build a **Millionaire Code** of behavior. For example, many professionals struggle with financial demands at work that conflict with financial dealings at home. We have counseled financial analysts who tested high on problem solving and certainly can do all the *right* analyses, at least for others. At home, they were spendthrift Pleasure Seekers. Problem solving was learned; they could put on the mask and go to work, but they were not going to attain a personal 3.5 Club membership. Their behavior and their personality were not congruent. While this combination of financial personalities makes for challenging thoughts, it is not unusual and suggestions throughout the rest of this book should spark personally satisfying ideas.

And it's certainly not unusual for opposites to attract, marry and wake up to the fact they see and value money differently. Because opposites attract they may regularly clash about money as well as the items that cash buys, such as a products they feel are necessary to meet inherent wants and needs. Each personality has desires and each individual approach can easily irk and perplex the other. In 2000, Olson and DeFrain surveyed 27,000 plus married couples about their financial personality and satisfaction with their mate's behavior with money. In their book, *Marriage in the Family*, they reported the results of their national study. Out of 27,000 couples, approximately 55,000 spouses, only 7,116 couples were happily married. More than two-thirds (69%) of the happy couples had no problem deciding how to spend and save money. Unfortunately, almost one-third *did* have trouble making decisions about cash management. While this may be common in the schema of a happily-ever-after marriage, it can cause stresses and strains in even the most prosperous marriages.

So, if the happy couples have problems with money, what about the unhappy ones? As you would expect, more than twice as many of those who are unhappy, specifically 74%, reported difficulties making financial management decisions. Obviously, when stresses from an unhappy marriage are present, financial personalities often work against any hopeful balance of cooperation. Of those couples having financial worries, half had problems budgeting and keeping records; the other half had problems managing credit cards and charge accounts.

There's also a peculiar twist worth mentioning. Whether you're married or single, happy or sad, data collected over the last decade further show that people fight about money regardless of how much they have. Felton-Collins noted this phenomenon in her 1990 book, *Couples and Money*. Fast forward to 2002, Bach noted and reported the same research results in *Smart Couples Finish Rich*. Personality impacts cash, and cash availability impacts behavior, specifically, the presence of personality strengths and weaknesses.

Arguments erupt because people have genuinely different views on cash flow. Opposites have trouble seeing eye-to-eye. After the bliss of the wedding, the limousine and honeymoon, a big spender may face their first personal experience with the bills if they are married to a big saver. For example, the new bride may be a security conscious Peacemaker linked with a happy-go-lucky Pleasure Seeker who now find themselves on the cash-merry-go-round-from-hell. But it doesn't have to be that way.

A large part of anyone's willingness to fight over money also depends on his or her core temperament. You are born with a core temperament, and you express it in your personality. It's personality that influences your instinct to spend or save, but you may not match your partner's. Character is what each of you do with these traits.

In fact, it's likely you and your spouse will face opposite views about money. Sometimes differing temperaments certainly add spice

---

Opposites Only Need To Think Of Concrete And Steel

Opposites can stay attracted and build a strong case for wealth development! As a matter of fact, all we need to do is look to the landscape architecture field for an example of opposites with material strengths and weaknesses that, when "partnered," build much stronger structures. Apparently, concrete on its own has what is called very high compressive strength. In other words, you can put a lot of weight on top of a large block of concrete, and it will not be crushed. However, concrete has very little tensile strength. If a long rectangular piece of concrete is laid across an opening and hit with a heavy weight it will crack and collapse.

On the other hand, steel has a very high tensile strength. If a long rectangular piece of steel is laid across an opening and hit with a heavy weight it will bend and spring back to its original shape or have a permanent bend. However, it will almost never crack. Steel does not have compressive strength. If a tall piece of unsupported steel is stood on end and a heavy weight is placed on top, it will likely bend and collapse.

When these two materials are combined in a product known as reinforced concrete, the result is a material that is far stronger than either concrete or steel. That is because the combination of these two has the strengths of both products, but does not have the weaknesses of either. The steel keeps the concrete from cracking, and the concrete keeps the steel from bending. This allows reinforced concrete to be used for beams carrying heavy weights over openings and columns supporting heavy weights.

A business partnership or a marriage can work in a similar way. As individuals, we all have strengths and weaknesses. Men and women have their own focus. Different families and cultures control money differently. Extroverts and introverts have their specific values. But if partners understand their different strengths and weaknesses, they can work together to combine their strengths to overcome many of their weaknesses. Consciousness precedes action!

---

to life; but if you don't understand where the other is coming from, the seasonings can leave a bitter taste.

So, a better way to view your interpersonal competing thoughts is to evaluate the unique financial strengths and weaknesses inherent in any relationship and apply the science behind the four financial **Millionaire Codes.** Whether you agree or disagree with your conscience or your spouse regarding money matters, if you understand where your "opposite" is coming from, you can develop a range of thoughts and together increase net worth. In addition to the age-old maxim "Know thyself," modern times require, "You better know your opposite, too." Consciousness precedes choosing the correct action to unlock behavioral codes.

To keep the peace and to help you both maximize your financial personality strengths, the following pages outline what can happen when Pleasure Seekers, Problem Solvers, Powerbrokers, and Peacemakers mix it up with their opposites.

One important note: Take heart, there are ways to work together on money and to solve the problems no matter how you view the subject. More help follows where we show how "blended Code families" can work positively together, too!

Problem Solvers With Pleasure Seekers

You took the quiz, and you discovered that you're a Problem Solver married to a Pleasure Seeker? Well, it makes for a creative contrast, a lot of guilty feelings, and a great deal of "You don't understand me." And, it's true. These two personalities are diametrically opposite. This means that they do not "naturally" see eye to eye. They will need to work on it. The Problem Solver is introverted, cultured, and scheduled, a planner who deals with and remembers the details. The opposite is the Pleasure Seeker who is outgoing, spontaneous, popular, and can't remember details worth a darn. They look and act like two characters in a popular TV sitcom.

Typically partners in any relationship — marriage or business — don't understand each other until they find common ground or understand where the other person is coming from. How will these partners function?

PLEASURE SEEKER STRENGTHS	PROBLEM SOLVER STRENGTHS
Talker	Listener, then is a
Spontaneous	Socratic questioner
Lively	Scheduled
Optimist	Cultured
Playful	Realist
Animated	Behaved
Dollar wise about prices	Orderly

Because Problem Solvers make perfectionist partners, they want everything in their world to be orderly, neat and clean. Is there anything wrong with an orderly checking account and savings plan, or sufficient insurance to shore up the inevitable event that follows Murphy's Law? No, these are strengths!

Because Pleasure Seekers are spirited promoters of fun, they want everything spontaneous, delightful, and demonstrative. They want their money to express their love and delight in people, in social events. Is there anything wrong with enjoying life, feeling comfortable with earnings and wanting to make more money to do better, or more fun things? No, these are their strengths!

But, what happens if a Problem Solver is shaken and stirred, but not satisfied — no matter the reason — with the current financial status? Their conscience is not clear. They will not settle for anything less than a clear conscience, and the partner who tries to change them will not find it easy. In a state of flux and insecurity, they are likely to withdraw and turn money worries inward (i.e., return to their *introverted* side) and become depressed. They are increasingly hard to please because of the challenge to their structured world. They need organized and neat homes, orderly long-range plans and financial order.

Trying to rein in the Pleasure Seeker with precision and order can be a difficult task. The more we try to structure and schedule their fun, the more unpredictable, undisciplined and brassy the Pleasure Seeker becomes. They can be loud, talkative, changeable and easily angered — the very opposite of their idealistic, thought-

PLEASURE SEEKER WEAKNESSES	PROBLEM SOLVER WEAKNESSES
Loud, extroverted	Withdrawn, introverted
Disorganized	Hard to please
Messy	Critical
Brassy	Bashful
Repetitious	Concrete thinker,
Show-off	specific with words
Permissive	Loner
Forgive and forget	Revengeful
Big spender	Unforgiving and never forgets

ful, self-sacrificing partner.

Problem Solvers inherently keep a record of wrongdoing simply because they need to track unsolved problems. They also have long memories and never forget. They are not necessarily out to get you (but they do have the evidence, and they keep it). They can tell you who, what, where, when and how someone mistreated them 20 years ago. They have a tendency to hold grudges. The Problem Solver limits change and spontaneity through silence and dependence on routines. They have (very) high ideals because their expertise lies in details. But this strength flips to weakness when they become obsessed, in other words, things are not *right* and must be fixed.

While the Problem Solver yearns for order, the Pleasure Seeker naturally creates disorder (but, unfortunately, rarely notices). The Pleasure Seeker promptly forgets about those records of wrongdoing, almost before the act is complete. Dependence on routine can make them seethe because they feel limited and controlled, which feels good to the Problem Solver. All strengths when taken to extremes can become weaknesses that seem almost intolerable to opposite financial codes of behavior.

To the Pleasure Seeker, the Problem Solver's introverted inertia is a conundrum. To the Problem Solver, the Pleasure Seeker's show-off, money-spending behavior is reprehensible and depressing. Perfectionist (Problem Solver) behavior toward money, so different from that of the Pleasure Seeker, just doesn't add up. For the Pleasure Seeker, the question remains "Why would someone want to take time to tidy up the house when the night is young?"

The "let's have fun" attitude is no match for the opposite attitude of "let's do things right." Furthermore, Pleasure Seekers party to forget their problems. Problem Solvers live to solve them, not forget them! They pride themselves on how perfectly they solved the problem, so don't hesitate to thank them for a job well done. Matter of fact, if you have a bone to pick with a perfectionist, think creatively about turning the question or the opportunity into a problem. For them, resolving chaos is pleasurable.

But watch out! Each day it's important to show each other that you are committed to the relationship in every conceivable way. Pleasure Seekers, be ready on time (we know, that's difficult). Mark birthdays and anniversaries on your calendar and make sure you personally pick out a gift that fits your partner's personality, not yours! Your Problem Solver partner values time, calendars, schedules and is very sensitive and thoughtful about traditions, and, while it may drive you crazy, this is good.

Turnabout is fair play. Problem Solvers, please, remain idealistic and resist getting depressed when the Pleasure Seeker is (irritatingly) optimistic. The Pleasure Seeker honestly sees the glass as always half-full, never half-empty. No clarification or logic on your part will change this perception. Their trait behaviors are not personally directed at you. They honestly have no desire to irritate or break down the relationship. They are on a mission to liven things up and make life fun.

Even sexual concordance in marriage is at risk when everything is taken personally. For example, it should not be an insult when the Pleasure Seeker is spontaneous, animated and sexually playful with their spouse. "Fun" and "fast" go along with their inherent strengths. Likewise, it should not be an insult when the Problem Solver wants more "romance," candlelight and the "right" music, which is often the opposite of "creative," "fun" or "fast."

THE PLEASURE SEEKER DESIRES...	BUT THE PROBLEM SOLVER THINKS...
Spontaneity, excitement Creative, enthusiastic sex Forgive and forget all trespasses (quickly!) Maximum flexibility and free response time	Spontaneous is not orderly, it's chaotic! Sex is romantic vs. creative (very different)! Automatically tracks problems that need fixes. Flexibility requires planning, scheduling.

Lucky is the spouse with a romantic perfectionist partner. Lucky, too, is the spouse with the demonstrative, playful, animated Pleasure Seeker!

Remember this maxim: Two people's strengths taken to extremes can work against each other. The Problem Solver's maximum need for order, planning and scheduling squashes the Pleasure Seeker's creativity. The Pleasure Seeker's jokes and money behaviors can appear to promote superficiality and instability. Their need for maximum flexibility can potentially lead to their inability to hear the problems — a bad mistake in the eyes of a good listener and Problem Solver. Spontaneity and excitement lead to the Pleasure Seeker's inattention to details and sensitivities, the latter being important to their opposite. Generally, when weaknesses multiply, the Problem Solver perceives that there is just too much play when there is so much work to do. But then the Pleasure Seeker perceives there is no more fun to be had!

So, if we can't change personality, we can change the way we see it. Here's how to do just that.

Problem Solver And Pleasure Seeker

Here's How To Capitalize On Millionaire Codes

Go back to the basics and think about what attracted you to each other. The Problem Solver probably thought it was great to be on the go with the Pleasure Seeker. After all, they have delightful ideas, and they can be so considerate of pleasing others. The Pleasure Seeker talks, and the Problem Solver listens — what a winning team.

In addition, they both are adventurers. The Pleasure Seeker looks for creative fun, while the Problem Solver can be quite the trekker and even enjoy being a daredevil. Originally we thought the daredevil trait was rare, but more and more observational data shows that the perfectionist is the best personality to organize, prepare and implement the details for a daring adventure. As long as the Pleasure Seeker does not run amuck being messy, inconsistent and forgetful (flip side of their strengths), and the Problem Solver does not control all spontaneity (flip side of their strengths), the combination of let's plan and schedule something new and exciting works great. This can be a highly compatible millionaire relationship.

Now, about money. Remember that most of the unhappy couples in trouble with money had problems budgeting and keeping records and half had problems managing credit cards and charge accounts. Most couples, happy and unhappy, struggle to get ahead. Guess which personality has the most problems managing credit cards and charge accounts? The Pleasure Seeker. They have the "shop til you drop" gene and compatible DNA (dollars, number, attitude). Who has trouble figuring out how to get ahead? The Problem Solver. Why? They over-plan for the future and over-worry about monetary security. They rarely get around to putting a plan in action. Who will budget and keep records? Naturally, the analytical, detail-oriented Problem Solver can. Who will self-monitor the charge cards? The Pleasure Seeker will promise to use credit for specific purchases only. So what is the problem? Assign tasks, right? It seems like a simple solution, and that's the one that most couples try first, but 99% of the time it just doesn't happen!

The Problem Solver often does not want to be involved. Why? Because they inherently know that they need to do it right. They want to feel accomplished in whatever field they are working in, so those tasks can be done perfectly. But that can take forever so they shy away from money management. Don't let them! They are valuable for the good job they will do. The Pleasure Seeker needs to work with the Problem Solver to appreciate attention to the details as well as the needs of the family.

The Pleasure Seeker, however, is the more creative of the two and has some tricks to make this project go faster. They need to be enlisted. However, reminders might be in order. Unfortunately, the Pleasure Seeker conveniently "forgets" they agreed with the Problem Solver to save for the future. They more easily stay focused on today. They forget how much they owe on charge cards and may think they can simply borrow from next month. Can the Pleasure Seeker slink away from financial management? No. They are the wealth creators of the partnership. But their problems with not valuing the future and charging into it (literally and figuratively) can lead to massive debt and bad credit. Like the old joke, the Pleasure Seeker just doesn't understand why the money is gone when they have more checks in their wallet. The Problem Solver sure does and is way too happy to explain why and then drones on about the screw-up for hours, maybe even weeks.

Ever notice how those pesky little credit card receipts grow while cash shrinks? If history in the relationship reflects an absence of order and stability, the credit charging lifestyle requires serious negotiation, and this will not be "fun." The Problem Solver senses a problem that needs a solution, one that the Pleasure Seeker wants to forget. While strict budgets can stress relationships, large debt on charge cards will stress both physical health and **Millionaire Codes**.

To summarize, Pleasure Seekers want to live for today and deal with tomorrow "some other time," if ever, because "tomorrow never really comes." They equate credit with cash; this does not create wealth — it destroys it. Credit cards are essentially a 21-day loan before big time fines and interest charges mount up. If current consumption is allowed to squash necessary investments for future success, the relationships cannot abide by **Millionaire Codes**.

Want to pick a bone with a Problem Solver about money?

It appears that when Pleasure Seeker spouses don't agree with Problem Solvers about money, the Problem Solver "has selective hearing." Need a suggestion on how to break through the barrier and get them to really hear you? If your Problem Solver has a private office at work, it pays to call them there, maybe even make a phone appointment. Don't lead off with a financial goal or a solution that seems clear to you but present the financial issue as a problem. After all, you are trying to communicate with Problem Solvers! They are "safe" in their office where they can shut the door and listen the same way they do when a client calls with a problem. Face to face confrontations with Problem Solvers, particularly family, do not always work because emotions add details that confuse the primary issue.

For instance, Pleasure Seekers and Powerbrokers tend to feel passionate about most issues, and they naturally communicate with more than words. Powerbrokers also use excitement and urgency, just what Problem Solvers hate and avoid! If you don't have the luxury of private offices, try scheduling aerobic walks after work where you can talk about the "tough" subjects and not be face to face. Then, be patient; the Problem Solver is a good listener if you break down the barriers to being heard.

Problem Solvers need to be included in tracking, planning for expenses and paying bills. Building wealth initially requires that order be paramount. A Problem Solver married to a Pleasure Seeker must be willing to step forward and meet the following responsibilities. (1) Review savings plans often and keep them in the forefront of the Pleasure Seeker's faulty memory. Don't try to trick the Pleasure Seeker into having savings. If the Pleasure Seeker perceives that money is being purposely withheld, they conclude that you don't care about them. Money means love, and no money means no love. (2) When order is established and financial goals for security are on track, the Problem Solver enjoys the status quo and will not seek change or growth. It is important to have financial growth to offset expenses and cope with faulty investments or economy. The Pleasure Seeker is the one to create financial opportunities. The Problem Solver needs to allow some instability in their stable world so that the Pleasure Seeker can satisfy some goals regarding moneymaking investments. Societies dominated by fearful perfectionists are never wealthy societies. Families are no different.

Occasionally doubters and fearful personalities are right, but most often they are not. Build up the Problem Solver's stamina for a reasonably comfortable degree of insecurity and instability but continue to review those investments that keep the family secure. Provide the Pleasure Seeker with creative tools, tapes and reading material that they *will use* to learn about finances, track expenses and goals.

Financial Traps To Avoid

The Pleasure Seeker's primary financial trap is living in the present and not planning for tomorrow	The Problem Solver's primary financial trap is requiring order when some chaos is inherent in growth.

The Problem Solver and the Powerbroker

These two personalities share both complimentary and compatible strengths. They are routinely considered to be very smart, even genius and most likely to succeed. Friends and family usually describe them as methodical organizers and "the" chiefs over memory retention. Consider the additional following trait strengths.

The Problem Solver sees the Powerbroker as a person who can "perfect" them. Where they are introverted, the Powerbroker is extroverted. Where they get bogged down in details to get things right, the Powerbroker comes along, digs them out and gets things done. Where they are economical, the Powerbroker knows just what to buy and when to buy it. They both like things to be right. They enjoy small numbers of close friends. They both value each other's intelligence quotient and terrific memories. There seems to be only one small hitch. The Powerbroker sets goals that the Problem Solver resents because deadlines often limit quality. But, it is a small price to pay for so many wonderful traits.

PROBLEM SOLVER STRENGTHS	POWERBROKER STRENGTHS
Introvert	Extrovert
Perfectionist (does less, but does it right)	Productive (does more, at any cost)
Idealistic	Goal oriented
Manager of details	Leader of big picture
Consistent, persistent organizer	Change agent who leads & organizes
Economical	End justifies the means (big spender)
Prefers small group of close friends	Prefers small group of close friends
Sensitive, wants things to be right	Must correct wrongs, is usually right
Precise memory for dates, details, genius	Memory of an elephant that never forgets

The Powerbroker recognizes that the Problem Solver values and needs their unique abilities — the ability to get things done and meet opposition head on when required. The Powerbroker allows the Problem Solver to handle details and envies their patience. But, not so fast! Where their strengths seem to compliment, their weaknesses are in direct contrast; and who doesn't lean toward some weaknesses some of the time?

When Murphy's Law prevails and situations go awry, the Powerbroker seeks to control for the sake of control and self worth. Dealings with money are no exception! In the meantime, the Problem Solver seeks control to shore up their sense of security. The controller criticizes "You are so irresponsible," while the controlled protests that "You treat me like a child."

The Problem Solver erroneously believes that they help *perfect* the Powerbroker; and no matter what, the Powerbroker believes they are the perfect one. These are illusory concepts of course but acted upon as truths. The Problem Solver thrives on cooperation, but they create opposition by revenging their partner's demanding nature, impatience, and their domination. If either one leads with their weaknesses, the other follows along.

PROBLEM SOLVER WEAKNESSES	POWERBROKER WEAKNESSES
Spends too much time planning	Demanding results, quickly
Deep need for approval	Rarely gives compliments or praise
Chooses difficult work; slow to get going	Chooses a challenge to remedy; Impatient
Revengeful (Silently)	Argumentative (Loud)
Hesitant to start projects	Can't relax (can't hesitate)
Emotional	Dislikes tears and emotions
Insecure	Dominates others, decides for them
Depressed over imperfections	Unsympathetic
Unforgiving	Can't say I'm sorry
Thrives on cooperation	Thrives on competition

Goals and checklists, schedules and time limits challenge the Powerbroker while they overwhelm their opposite. The Problem Solver expects everyone to value quality over quantity. Identifying details, having sufficient time to plan and organize challenges the Problem Solver. However, too much planning and lack of deadlines overwhelm their opposite. They make the Powerbroker feel powerless who in turn tries to spin the goals back into high speed and expects loyalty to their purpose, which make the Problem Solver powerless.

Problem Solver and Powerbroker

Here's How to Capitalize on Millionaire Codes

We've said this before, and it's worth saying again. All relationships have trouble with money, but unhappy relationships have a great deal of trouble with money. Most couples, happy and unhappy, struggle to get ahead. Powerbrokers never met a plan to develop riches they didn't like — unless it's one that's slow, long term and mitered with details. Budgeting and record keeping need to be left to the Problem Solver. The Problem Solver, on the other hand, sees no value in trying to accomplish something worthwhile without sufficient time, organization and details. They manage best but can take a leadership role by identifying funds that they turn over to the Powerbroker to power up.

Powerbrokers naturally compete with themselves or with others, whoever is first in line at the time. They need money to compete and often forget to cooperate — actually, they don't forget, it does not come naturally. Taking control of self is good; however, being possessive and taking control of others will slowly and surely destroy **Millionaire Codes**. Controlling a Problem Solver without respect for their need for security and order will backfire. Because poor results play out slowly, the Powerbroker is fooled into thinking that a greater push will accelerate goals. As a result, they often fail to recognize inherent risks; they keep on keeping on; throw good money after bad; and, simply put, have trouble walking away and cutting their losses. Their loss challenges their ego, and that's not a good thing.

The Problem Solver, on the other hand, listens to complaints and is often willing to stay in the background seeking to resolve those issues. Then, if things are still not quite right, they avenge the misbehavior. Competition is not inherent unless they learned it at home. They naturally cooperate. They do not want to compete for resources, stability, security or finances. When pushed to compete, they often nit-pick over every action and passive-aggressively create inaction. Meanwhile, money is either held in limbo or evaporates as a result of the stalemate between who wins and who gives in.

In marriages, money can be a scapegoat for other issues that seem too difficult to resolve. When leaning toward perfectionist weaknesses, revengeful behaviors can include hiding large sums of money to satisfy a need for more security. Or, Problem Solvers may find it is easier to worry about money than to diagnose "why" they haven't had sex with their spouse in the last month. In so many ways they're far more intensely focused on their purpose, opportunities, and ventures than they are about their sexual prowess.

To summarize, the Problem Solver often needs a push to compete, and the Powerbroker needs a pull to cooperate. Both must shift their mindset where money is concerned. The Powerbroker is a wealth creator; the Problem Solver is the wealth manager. One naturally leads; the other naturally manages. This is good! Each values planning for the future, but one has a shorter, quicker definition of when the future is expected to arrive. The Problem Solver thinks long term — very long term — about retirement; the Powerbroker plans six months out. Both financial plans are **Millionaire Codes**. Building on and combining codes is a winning approach but remember one personality is the big spender, and one is the big saver. If this obvious fact is ignored, it becomes a secret wealth blaster. Communication about wants and needs for power, control and security is critical. Defining what money means *personally* is not taboo. Secrets are taboo. The Powerbroker will create wealth assuming they cooperate with the Problem Solver to track, monitor and manage the details.

Financial Traps To Avoid

The Problem Solver's primary financial trap is requiring order when disorder is prevalent in growth	The Powerbroker's primary financial trap is thriving on competition when cooperation is needed

The Problem Solver and the Peacemaker

Two introverted financial personalities can create a perfectly peaceful lifestyle. Pushy salesmen have a hard time cracking **The Millionaire Code** for these two. While the Problem Solver is serious and purposeful, the Peacemaker is easygoing and relaxed. They value function over fun. The Peacemaker's motto is "Be careful, don't look for problems." The Problem Solver sees problems before they are apparent, worries and then seeks to solve the

PROBLEM SOLVER STRENGTHS	PEACEMAKER STRENGTHS
Introvert	Introvert
Perfectionist	Everything's fine;
Idealistic	"whatever," adaptable
Manager of details,	Peaceful and agreeable
slow and steady	Management abilities,
Finds the right way	slow and steady
Economical	Find the easy way
Prefers small group	Born saver; prefers
of close friends	financial shelters
Sensitive, wants things	Many friends
to be right	Compassionate and concerned
Precise memory for dates,	Sensitive, Natural mediator
details, genius	Competent and steady
Often moved to tears with	Natural historian
compassion	

PROBLEM SOLVER WEAKNESSES	PEACEMAKER WEAKNESSES
Spends too much time worrying, planning	Prefers watching money, slow & safe
Deep need for approval	judgmental (but a good
Chooses difficult work;	listener)
slow to get going.	Chooses the easy way;
Revengeful	hard to get moving.
Hesitant to start projects	Quiet will of iron
Emotional	Lazy, resists change,
Worrier	resents being pushed
Perfectionist; economical	Sarcastic,
Can be depressed	Teasing then uninvolved
Unforgiving	Insecure
	Cheap, wants the easy,
	comfortable life
	Nonchalant
	Avoids responsibility

problems early. An examination of strengths shows how compatible these two can be.

Problem Solvers and Peacemakers are compassionate and content with economical lifestyles. Both are inherently good at managing dollars, numbers and attitudes (DNA). Neither has an inclination to risk money for growth and neither cares. These two financial personalities are compatible; slow and steady wins the race. However, it is highly recommended that this team find a certified financial planner to counter and keep perspective on their weaknesses.

Essentially, they have the potential to be two worrywarts and then blame each other. If the situation goes too far without verbal communication (which is likely), the Peacemaker presents a quiet will of iron, unbendable even in the face of revenge. It is a standoff. If they are able to talk, problems end up as worries for the Problem Solver who gets easily depressed over imperfections. The

Peacemaker dampens the expression of any emotion. Nothing changes, which is to their liking; but nothing is resolved or really peaceful either, which irks both. Neither can get a project up and going, but if someone else will start it (like an outsider), one of them will manage it, albeit with a grumble or two.

Problem Solver And Peacemaker

Capitalize On Millionaire Code

What's their approach to money? Remember Olson found that most couples, happy and unhappy, struggle to get ahead, but who drives this partnership to get ahead? Neither. Who in this relationship will run up credit card debt? Neither, if they play to their strengths. Who will budget and keep records? Neither one will, unless the Problem Solver reluctantly agrees to take responsibility. They need the financial information to calm worries and to solve problems. If left to their own devices, the Peacemakers will never get around to it. The Peacemaker unconsciously knows that where problems are embraced, new responsibilities are close behind. The Problem Solver likes to solve problems, and the Peacemaker doesn't want to hear about them. This leaves the problem solver without emotional support for their imperfect financial plan; but, at least, the Peacemaker will have concern and be compassionate.

This partnership needs a financial overseer, and the reasons are twofold. First, the Problem Solver requires predictable order in financial records, sometimes to the point of holding the line where investments don't even cover normal expenses and inflation. In other words, they get back less than they put into investments because any chaos in the stock or real estate markets is imperfect and depressing.

Second, the Peacemaker prefers the peace of mind and status they feel when their monies are readily visible in accessible accounts like money markets and certificate of deposits. They also want to keep the peace at all costs and throughout the family. This personality will do almost anything to help a needy family member, even abandon long-range, secure financial plans in lieu of one individual's immediate need. While it is commendable to help needy

Financial Traps To Avoid

The Problem Solver's primary financial trap is to demand order when disorder is essential to growth.	**The Peacemaker's primary financial trap is to drop routine financial commitments in favor of keeping the peace with a hurting person in need.**

family members, loaning without clear expectation of repayment jeopardizes both financial wealth building and personal relationships. Remember the Problem Solver plans their budget and will understandably resent the financial intruder. The next person in line for resentment is the loaner. Too much of anything is no good. Renegotiate how to handle family loans. For instance, you could just decide on gifting a specific amount or elect to draw up a contract for repayment, spelling out interest, payment schedules.

In general, build in some room for chaos and put some monies into investments that earn compounded interest and cannot be easily tapped or drained.

The Powerbroker and the Peacemaker

The Powerbroker equates money with self-control, independence, self-worth; and the Peacemaker equates money with comfortable status and peace of mind, seemingly very compatible needs. While the end appears to justify the means, we can appreciate how different their ways and means are when we examine their strengths.

The Powerbroker sees the Peacemaker as the good listener, smart, and submissive (if not subordinate) to their leadership and goals; and that's okay with the Peacemaker. The Peacemaker prefers to watch while the Powerbroker leads, so all appears right with their world. They are both good in emergencies. The

POWERBROKER STRENGTHS	PEACEMAKER STRENGTHS
Extroverted & outspoken	Introverted listener,
Productive, moves quickly	holds back responses
to action	Calm, cool, collected,
Goal oriented	slow to take action
Leader of big picture	Submissive
Change agent who leads	Peaceful and agreeable
& organizes	Management skills,
Finds the fast way	watches and judges
Creates wealth; end justifies	Finds the easy way
the means	Bigger saver;
Has Little need for lots	prefers safe shelters
of friends	Many friends,
Must correct wrongs,	easy to get along with
is usually right	Natural mediator,
Excels in emergencies	everybody is right
Tenacious	Competent & steady,
	good under pressure
	Inoffensive

Powerbroker moves fast, and the Peacemaker looks for the easy way, succumbing as soon as the Powerbroker finds the way. If they are so lucky to be wealthy by Peacemaker's definition, money issues will not be a problem. Together, they represent the biggest spender and the biggest saver, but the Peacemaker only values a consistent and balanced life. As long the goals don't involve them and they enjoy a consistent and balanced life, all's fair in love and war. War only arises when both parties exercise their weaknesses.

When weaknesses prevail, the Powerbroker sees the Peacemaker as their project. They will set goals to motivate the Peacemaker, set deadlines to get things moving, and probably end up deciding for them too. The Peacemaker stays uninvolved, watching, waiting, and expecting to be bullied. However, the fireworks start when the Peacemaker resists change because that

POWERBROKER WEAKNESSES	PEACEMAKER WEAKNESSES
Adheres to goals, demands achievement	Not goal oriented, lacks self-motivation
Dominates	Lazy, careless, resists
Impatient, decides for others	change and demands Indifferent to plans;
Argumentative, passionate	Hard to get moving Dampens enthusiasm
Can't relax	and passion
May be rude or tactless	Lazy and resents being pushed Quiet will of iron
Knows everything (and it's not funny!)	Sarcastic, teasing with dry wit Fearful, doubting, worrier,
Unsympathetic	needs sympathy
Has expensive taste	Cheap!
Demands loyalty	Nonchalant
Can do everything perfectly	Avoids responsibility, so ...you do it!

upsets their need for balanced and contented lifestyle. It's as if one moves on the fast tract while the other is laid back in the slow lane. One likes expensive things, and the other prefers "cheap" or respectfully stated, "inexpensive." Can this relationship be saved? Only when the Powerbroker realizes how much subtle power the Peacemaker has (and not so subtle when they use the "silent treatment") do they begin to begrudgingly cooperate.

Powerbroker And Peacemaker

How To Capitalize On Millionaire Codes

We've said it before, but we need to remind each duo. Most couples, happy and unhappy, struggle to get ahead. In this relationship, who will have problems keeping records, managing credit cards and budgeting? The Powerbroker, definitely. The

Peacemaker would rather starve than run out of cash or build up a credit bill that cannot be cleared in 21 days.

Who will get this partnership moving ahead? The Powerbroker can do it. They never met a plan to develop riches that they did not like. The Peacemaker will typically be unconcerned about building great wealth just as long as there is enough money to pay bills and feel secure, maybe even "high on the hog," which is the Powerbroker's goal and plan. Peacemakers will be amiable, patient and inoffensive *as long as* the plan works.

Sometimes Peacemakers try to intervene when they see things moving very fast. They inherently want to slow things down. They prefer and feel safer with a slower pace, one that brings peace. While involvement is good when security is shored up, letting them take control can send wealth management down the tubes. The reason is common sense. They value an even keel, balanced lifestyle; and they think their Powerbroker partner will be much happier when, they too, slow down. This is just one of those times when they do know what's best for them but can't see what the other needs. They see a distinct difference between the fast tract and the peace-of-mind tract. If the Peacemaker senses the fast tract financial plan is off kilter, then status and peace of mind is interrupted. They will exert a quiet will of iron, which may be what the Powerbroker finds distasteful, and will never admit that is what is needed. Obviously, a lack of money is a direct affront to each person's self-respect and peace of mind.

To summarize, if these two partners scored high on these traits (both primary personalities), they are diametrically opposite. What does this mean? It means that these two partners have fewer traits in common than most other relationships. They don't "naturally" see eye-to-eye and will have to work on it and communicate clearly. The Powerbroker is typically on the fast track to grow money while the Peacemaker is on the slow and easy path to maintain the status quo. Too much of anything is no good, and the Powerbroker's desire for competition will often squelch the Peacemaker's thirst for cooperation. In contrast, the Peacemaker highly values helping family and friends out whenever possible, no

Financial Traps To Avoid

The Powerbroker's primary financial trap is inherently competing when the situation calls for cooperation	The Peacemaker's primary financial trap is succumbing to extended family/friends' needs over more personal needs.

matter how much their partner is inconvenienced or their goals interrupted. This can ignite like gunpowder. Neither will easily understand why each other acts the way they decide to do.

The Pleasure Seeker And The Peacemaker

Again we have an extroverted talker with an introverted listener, a popular combination, but not one without significant differences and honest disagreements. The Pleasure Seeker is on

PLEASURE SEEKER STRENGTHS	PEACEMAKER STRENGTHS
Extroverted talker, witty storyteller	Introverted listener with quick, dry wit
Spontaneous	Adaptable
Lively	Peaceful and agreeable
Optimist	Pessimist but avoids conflicts
Finds the fun way	Find the easy way
Money means fun and ways to show love	The biggest saver; prefers financial shelters
Loves many friends, fun to get along with	Has many friends, natural mediator
Playful	Easy to get along with
Animated	Competent and steady
Physically holds on to listeners	Compassionate listener
Emotional and demonstrative	Calm, cool and collected

PLEASURE SEEKER WEAKNESSES	PEACEMAKER WEAKNESSES
Bigger spender	Bigger saver; prefers watching
Loud	money
Disorganized	Judgmental
Messy	Hard to get moving, resents
Brassy	being pushed
Repetitious	Straight-laced,
Show-off	Quiet will of iron
Permissive with money;	Lazy, resists change
falls fast for sales	Sarcastic
Forgive and forget	Quiet worrier
Money-What's	Cheap
responsibility	Nonchalant
got to do with it?	Avoids responsibilities;
	problems only disrupt peace
	in the valley

the fun track, and the Peacemaker wants self-respect, comfortable financial status and peace of mind.

The Pleasure Seeker naturally loves everyone, but especially those folks who love their jokes, stories and physical signs of affection. The Peacemaker fits right in there — compassionate listeners with a periodic, dry wit that can crack up a Pleasure Seeker. The fact that they don't need much money initially seems perfect to the Pleasure Seeker who needs no help in finding ways to spend money. The problem comes with financial personality goals. Examine the weaknesses of each in the table above.

It really never enters the mind of a Pleasure Seeker to *hold* onto money for peace of mind. They find that boring. They want to enjoy life, be loved and love others. It's a special pleasure when others reciprocate their affection (Hint: It usually takes some money). What is the problem with that? Nothing, unless strengths are taken to extremes. For instance, the Pleasure Seeker is not going to please their opposite if they do *not* want to save for a rainy day, plan for tomorrow, "watch" (this is a favorite word for their opposite partner) their money grow slowly on the vine. Then their Peacemaker partner becomes NO FUN, spoils their party, and rains on their parade! As a result, each one is very likely to be dumbfounded by the other's behavior. "How can you think like that?" is a common question that comes up in the surveys. The only answer that Popeye gave Olive Oil, "I am who I am." So, can this financial relationship be saved? Absolutely!

Pleasure Seeker-Peacemaker Partnerships

Capitalizing On Their Millionaire Codes

From the start of their relationship, each will have to work at leaning toward their strengths and listening when the other sends up smoke signals that can be easily misunderstood. Many a philosopher has suggested that happiness is made up of three elements: something to love, something to do and something to look forward to. Think through and communicate what these three elements mean as priorities.

For example, the Peacemaker's priorities may very well vary around a theme. Element #1: Something to love is their partner, but there are additional joys to love. Needless to say, raising happy children and financially securing all educational journeys are goals. Element #2: Something to do is likely securing a "comfortable" home with "comfortable" furnishings. We have it from the finest authorities — our clients — that a recliner or comfy chair is required and they look forward to watching TV and holding hands. Element #3: Something to look forward to might be having "money in the bank." Needless to say, zero accessible dollars and mounting debt hardly fits the bill for the Peacemaker.

While the Pleasure Seeker is likely to share those items on the "something to love" list, they love "something to look forward to" or wish lists. The Pleasure Seeker is the expert advisor for this list! Never confuse wants and needs with the Pleasure Seeker. Keep the list focused on "to do" events in immediate future, vacations, birthdays and holidays. Some Pleasure Seekers can visualize a year's worth but most eyes glaze over after 3-5 events. Stay with planning "events" because it is difficult to visualize months ahead. "Tomorrow" is a foreign concept — it needs to have a fun anchor, like an event. Put "needs" on "something to do lists," not "wish lists." Admit it, you know this personality and they won't remember where they left those lists anyway. But they can appreciate that the wish lists are in the trusty hands of the Peacemaker. Include with "the wish list" a budget for each event based on the family's ability to pay. The Pleasure Seeker wins when the couple can bring the plan out in advance of spending for a memory refresher — less to discuss and they can move into action. The Peacemaker wins by stabilizing financial status, by getting grounded, and getting a commitment to save up in order to address the wish lists. You have your special event and wish list budget in tow!

We have given you some tips for communicating about finances, expenses and budgets with Pleasure Seekers. Here are three suggestions for communicating with the Peacemaker: (1) Review the test results with your partner, specifically, opposite traits, wants, needs. (2) Compromise and communicate! (3) In order to communicate with the Peacemaker, Littauer suggested in her book *Getting Along with Almost Anybody* that you study Japanese – honestly! In Japan, people learn to ask questions that elicit positive answers. A negative answer makes both parties feel bad. Feeling bad is to be avoided. So, when the Peacemaker's mother-in-law has come to stay, instead of asking if the guest bedroom will *ever* be available again in your lifetime, ask if you can plan to move your office equipment in next week or at the beginning of the month. Make the choices reasonable and ones

Financial Traps To Avoid

Pleasure Seekers financial trap is to get caught up in today believing we can't live "tomorrow" today.	**The Peacemaker's primary financial trap is making peace in crisis with one individual and postponing peace with family plans.**

that you can live with, even be happy with, and then expect a
workable response, one from your partner's strengths.

The Pleasure Seeker And The Powerbroker

Two extroverts, how refreshing — great fun, just alike, right?
Except, …they compete for money, for the chance to talk, for the
attention of an audience. They expect each other to remain optimistic, regardless. How does this relationship build wealth (or
do they)?

PLEASURE SEEKER STRENGTHS	POWERBROKER STRENGTHS
Extroverted talker, storyteller	Extroverted, outspoken
Spontaneous	Goal oriented
Lively	Productive
Optimist; sees the big picture	Leads the big picture
Finds the fun way	Change agent who finds the
Money means fun and ways	fast way
to show love	Money means power, control
Loves many friends,	Likes cohesive group of
fun to get along with	friends
Playful, affectionate	Gets down to work
Animated	Unaffectionate
Physically holds on to	Daring
listeners	Must correct wrongs,
Emotional, demonstrative;	is usually right
short memory	Great memory;
	they never forget

They enjoy each other's company and seem so much alike, on
the same page, with the same ideals — until you put them under
a microscope. The Powerbroker sets goals that the Pleasure Seeker
brushes off. Goals, plans and schedules tend to supplant spontaneous play for the Pleasure Seeker. The Powerbroker is the ultimate change agent, but the Pleasure Seeker often tires of change

PLEASURE SEEKER WEAKNESSES	POWERBROKER WEAKNESSES
Doesn't analyze details	Doesn't analyze details
The big spender	Big spender
Loud, directive and impatient	Loud, directive and impatient
Disorganized, loves trivia, games	Organized; Bored with trivia
Messy	Demands order, achievement
Brassy	Impatient, decides for others
Repetitious	Little tolerance for mistakes
Show-off	Can't relax
Permissive	Dominates and is argumentative
Fickle and forgetful	May be rude or tactless
Makes excuses	Rremembers!
	Knows everything

if it doesn't culminate in fun. The Powerbroker wants to get down and work. The Pleasure Seeker wants to get down and play. The Pleasure Seeker cannot remember wrongs committed (much less their own); and the Powerbroker needs, nay, demands to right those wrongs. Unfortunately for the Pleasure Seeker, the Problem Solver is usually right about those wrongs. So, what happens when they face off? Weaknesses kick in.

Weaknesses become a real problem when it comes to love and money. Remember the Powerbroker is the only one of these two who foresees the future. The Pleasure Seeker tends to deny it will ever appear. Unless money is abundant now, and into the foreseeable future, the Powerbroker will push to exercise their plans to raise available money. After all, money equals cash, credit, savings, other people's money, and, of course, stock options, futures and whatever other ideas accountants can entice them with. The Pleasure Seeker never has a plan …get the picture? What is left for the Pleasure Seeker? Remnants.

The Pleasure Seeker can and will get offensive or even physically ill, anxious or depressed, if they lose all control over money, have no input into where the money is going and, worst of all, and/or have no money to spend. Just because they are not scheduled planners, they are not incompetent with money! Because the Pleasure Seeker is spontaneous, learns quickly and understands other's wants and needs, this personality is extremely successful in education, stock or real estate ventures. After a quick and accurate read of client needs, they can locate and sell you "the" perfect property, the perfect insurance policy, the perfect pool — how about a new cell phone plan!

The Problem Solver, on the other hand, is more directed, impatient, organized and generally more focused to land *a* deal. They cinch deals with dollars, numbers and facts — ones that cannot be reasonably argued. Obviously, this is not the only wealth scenario, but a capital investment strategy we often hear from experience.

Pleasure Seekers and Powerbrokers

Capitalizing on their Millionaire Codes

When it comes to their handling money together, remember half of the unhappy couples in trouble with money had problems budgeting and keeping records, and the other half had problems managing credit cards and charge accounts. Most couples, happy and unhappy, struggle to get ahead. Who will drive this partnership to get ahead? They both can but as you will see, it's up to each personality's creativity!

It can be argued that both personalities define money in similar ways. Both are extroverted personalities who want and need money for their personal definition of control, power and, ostensibly, fun, even if specific visions differ. So how can they use their individual, yet similar **Millionaire Codes**? They must get out of each other's way!

The Powerbroker can choose either to compete or not with the Pleasure Seeker for money. The way we see it, Powerbrokers have a choice: (1) to come together and agree or (2) to contend, struggle, and argue. Only the individual personality can choose. Competition involves planning, organized implementation and, strategically speaking, either cooperation or contention. Choosing contention can be synonymous with combativeness, rivalry, battles and litigation, the most damaging to your **Millionaire Code**. Choosing *cooperation* is synonymous with *association, alliance and partnership*. Too often the Powerbroker does not think that it is brave to cooperate, but cooperation is usually the definition of success. So which do you want, agree or argue? It is a personal choice, perhaps even a pre-wired one.

The Powerbroker does not need to challenge the Pleasure Seeker's definition of the future. Synonymous for *future*, at least as a verb, is *to look forward, anticipate, and expect*, traits that really mean something fun to the Pleasure Seeker. So while they can't live in the future, they do a darn good job of getting excited, planning for all sunny days, and looking forward to something. They can honestly feel disoriented when the future means "coming years," so don't go there. Stay in the "present" future.

Actually, the opposite of future is futureless, having no prospect of future success, and that would not be a good thing for Pleasure Seekers. The way we see it, Pleasure Seekers, like Powerbrokers, have a choice: Deny that they love to anticipate and look forward to success (thereby, spend it now!) or cooperate in developing and implementing plans for the near future.

To summarize, both personalities have financial success fever flowing in their veins. As a result, they may not take the time to listen to the wants and needs of the other. The Pleasure Seeker struggles to live in the here and now, spontaneously and energetically. The Powerbroker struggles to purposely pursue a goal where the end justifies the means. But watch out! Something is missing — the details.

Financial Traps To Avoid

The Pleasure Seeker's financial trap is living it up for today and resolving to borrow for tomorrow	The Powerbroker's primary financial trap is capitalizing on competitive strengths when cooperation is the balance needed.

Millionaire Code Stories

Today And Tomorrow Find Love At Last:
Pleasure Seeker (Big Spender) And
Problem Solver (Big Saver) Use Millionaire Codes

Jessica and Mark are married, in their early 30s and scored exactly opposite on the money personality test. Jessica came out high in the "live for today" category (big spender Pleasure Seeker), and Mark scored high on the "live for tomorrow" paradigm (big saver Problem Solver). Mark had been a saver all his life and never saw it as a burden. He naturally focused on setting aside money for some-time in the future. Jessica, on the other hand, always harbored a notion of sweeping her husband away from the day-to-day grind, maybe leading travel groups through exotic cities.

Until that future day comes, there is today and tomorrow. They had just bought their first house, a cottage that Jessica said needed cosmetic surgery and a lot of furniture. Mark, on the other hand, was fretting over the new mortgage, homeowner's insurance, umbrella coverage, health and now life insurance (since they have debt), saving for incidentals (like roofs, car repairs) as well as maxing out their tax-deferred savings plans. Their disposable income took a sizeable hit and shrunk. Jessica felt deprived!

After discovering her **Millionaire Code**, Jessica decided she did not want the responsibility of managing their money. Mark realized he was too much of a perfectionist to take the lead when he had such a big learning curve ahead of him. Working with an adviser, they ventured, would make them think more realistically.

The adviser charged Jessica with the laborious task of compiling the many details of their financial lives. Regardless of personality, they both scored low on risk tolerance, having seen what the recession of 2000 did to their parents' and siblings' reserves. They wanted to retain the modest amount they made so they only agreed to 50% stocks. They can re-evaluate later when they get more comfortable and Jessica is "less deprived." She says she does feel better, a) being finished with the incredibly boring tasks, b) having learned a little about the complex processes needed for wealth preservation, and c) knowing Mark feels more financially secure. Mark does feel better and clearer of purpose. "Today," the priority is to stabilize their monthly income and outgo with so many new responsibilities. He has Jessica on his side. She can do her homework for the seriously important tasks of keeping costs down for furniture by scouring sales and local flea markets. Maybe, just maybe, "tomorrow" will be the right time to buy.

Ellie and Paul shake loose their financial traps.

Ellie was the most likely to succeed Powerbroker, and Paul the Problem Solver was smitten. First comes love, then marriage, two children and problems galore. That was when Ellie started wondering if they were going to be destitute. The reason was that Paul was still making the same amount of money after the 2nd child that he was making before the first. Wanting more money, nice clothes, piano lessons for kids, she took in sewing dresses for special events. She was an expert seamstress and enjoyed a nice salary! But as time got short with kids and other responsibilities, she could not increase her sewing to match her wants and needs. While she had savings, she could not make ends meet with just cash flow. She was pretty sure she had exhausted her control over time and money. This is not good for Powerbrokers.

Paul owned his own business. The big auto parts businesses were moving in and clients could get cheaper pricing with big over small businessmen. Paul was not adventuresome, hated change and was grateful for the security that he mustered in small circles. He was very concerned about Ellie choosing money as her challenge to remedy. He had personal reasons for not doing anything but Ellie was unsympathetic and impatient. They could not change each other; they could only change themselves. And this is what Ellie decided to do.

Ellie got her real estate license, not to be an agent, but to buy up small properties and fix them up for rental. She studied and surveyed properties, invested her savings from sewing and started small with one rental while the kids were in school. In the afternoons, the kids joined her, helped, raked, swept, painted, and cleaned a growing number of properties. She cornered a market of college-age renters. Seeing that they rarely, if ever, had furniture, she took some profits and started going to estate sales. She picked up some very nice pieces of furniture for the houses, and now she and the kids had more jobs they could do together — finish furniture. Interestingly, she soon developed a market for selling the furniture she finished and was able to purchase more upscale pieces — and save big. She finally sold all the rentals, all the furniture she did not want, capitalized on tax savings and retired a wealthy woman — who comfortably supported

Paul (in the manner to which he got accustomed). If you
can't change personality, change the eyes that see it.

Will they or won't they? That is the question.

Marjorie and Sam have been married 25 years with two grown
sons. Marjorie had the intuitive Problem Solver DNA and was very
successful at preparing corporate tax reports while the boys were
growing up. Sam was a Peacemaker, a 20 year veteran manager over
hundreds of employees in a large corporation. Sam has always been
hard to get moving with money. That seemed logical while the family
was growing and securing education for the boys.

They had been big savers and were in excellent shape with an
impressive retirement and pension. They had held the financial
reigns so readily accessible savings were substantive. So what was the
problem? Everything from all angles was covered, and Sam would not
talk about spending money on dreams. Marjorie kept talking about
kitchen remodeling, about a vacation, and asking what would he
want. Sam did not respond — "uh-huh" and "that would be nice"
went on and on and on. Marjorie went from looking for the "right"
way to spend "a little" to needing Sam's approval for anything, and
then, you guessed it, to expressing revenge. She was moving to
France! She retired from her job, made intricate and daredevil plans
to live and adventure out from one city. Sam could join her or not. He
didn't, and she didn't, but she got his attention and remodeled the
kitchen.

Ann vs. Ron — And the Winner is...

Fortunately, a Powerbroker wife and Peacemaker husband finally
learned where each of their strengths were located and put their
consciousness to action, pencil to the paper, and money where their
mouth was!

Ann handles the money and day-to-day financial management;
Ron does the research and makes the investment decisions. They
discuss major purchases and other money decisions. They have always
believed in living below their means, although they haven't always
agreed on how far below that should be! There's the problem.

The Peacemaker, Ron, can be naturally critical about spending
money. Ron is cool, reserved, and objective. The Peacemaker just
smiles and postpones acting on any expense by nodding or saying
"no." Ann, the Powerbroker just keeps talking, sure that she will hit

on the magical words that will incite action. She gets frustrated when she perceives that Ron is indifferent about making plans to spend money. He is. She thinks she can talk him into the house repair or investment or purchase. She is wrong. The Peacemaker counts on her running out of words. The end result? They don't fix up their house as much as she wants, and they don't stash all monies under the mattress like he wants.

For Ron, things just need to be "good enough." He is most concerned about watching, taking care of the money. Ann generally dislikes planning, monitoring long-range retirement goals in minute detail. Ron thrives on that and prides himself on thinking concretely about budgets, priorities and savings. Ann is a passionate person who enjoys fantasizing about grand schemes and the way the two of them can express their creativity and potential with their money. We know from research that personality is impervious to sex differences. But, boy (and girl) do we express ourselves differently in relationships. Why? Emotions! Multiple research studies have reported a strong gender component to emotional memory. Women remember emotion-laden events more deeply and vividly than do men, and they use different parts of their brains when doing so

When women passionately express their feelings about money, men, stop what you're doing and listen up. Men, the debate will not go away. It may move off that one subject you don't want talk about, but the debate just shifts. The Peacemaker can be unenthusiastic about spending money. When they exercise their quiet will of iron, are reticent and self-righteous about what's not important (their judgment call), they are working in their weaknesses. This couple knew they had different money personalities before marriage, but as Ann says, "I realize now what money means to a person and that it really does motivate their actions, decisions and attitudes toward a lot of things in life."

Ron is watching while Ann researches the big picture for a balanced portfolio of investments and savings. He promises to enthusiastically listen for opportunities he can live with. Ann meanwhile promises to remember Ron's need for a solid financial status.

Pleasure Seeker Meets Peacemaker:
Can This Relationship Be Saved?

Carol, a Pleasure Seeker, is one of two partners in her own law firm. She enjoys the practice of law, loves talking to clients on the phone, and keeps up enriching relationships. She expects to get paid well for 50+ hour weeks and the headaches of administering a ten-person staff. Her partner, Brenda, is her opposite — a Peacemaker with money. She wants and needs high earnings for respect, status and peace of mind. She demands it and good for her!

Because Brenda demands a safe way to hold on to principal, she's a typical "mattress stuffer." Financial advisors define mattress stuffers as folks who put all money in money markets, certificates of deposit or government bonds. Brenda watches her money in a couple of high profile stocks, a very conservative profit sharing plan, CDs and a money market account. Her knowledge about finances is typically sufficient to satisfy peace of mind. She can even sound like a guru about stocks and P/E ratios. Her "saving style," however, often does not match the rate of inflation, but principal is safe. Regarding inflation and planning for retirement, she "will get around to it someday."

Carol wanted to make some changes — a given and a constant for Pleasure Seekers! She debated how to accommodate Brenda's slow and easy "better safe than sorry" DNA. She anticipated indifference and resentment but wanted to grow the firm. Unfortunately, she knew full well that making changes and adding responsibilities are threats for the Peacemaker! Brenda had gotten quite comfortable with the status quo of the 1990's. Carol had been accommodating; however, work on new cases was piling up. Brenda did not like the different kind of cases and, silently — a Peacemaker, passive-aggressive strategy — she refused to work on them. Carol needed to address the lack of productivity in the office but dreaded the negative, pessimistic and analytical response she knew she'd receive when she just wanted to get the work done.

Brenda had an excuse for everything! She had been getting in later and later, complaining of exhaustion, sinus and allergy problems. Carol confronted Brenda, noting that she was coming in by 11:00, basically in time for lunch and working on selected cases while pressing matters went unattended. Presenting this as a problem brought out the worst in Brenda. This financial personality is not a Problem Solver! Working in their weaknesses, they have a critical but self-righteous, quiet will-of-iron surrounding money issues. For instance, when faced with the lack of productivity, specifically regarding partnership responsibilities, she refused new purchases or upgrades in software and other equipment to accommodate additional work. She would not approve hiring additional lawyers, and she rejected any additional clerical help. What is a Pleasure Seeker to do?

Typically, opposite personalities attract and cycle through a period of "de-attraction." Time passed, marked by decreased billings and increased client complaints. Carol was ready to address the root problems of financial personality conflicts. Carol had to borrow some traits from the Peacemaker, namely (1) prioritize change, (2) be competent and steady, at peace with available choices, (3) be good under pressure and listen carefully for the easy way. Carol presented a strong case and the seriousness of the situation set in. Brenda recognized there was work to do and billings to realize.

Partnerships are serious relationships, and this one was heading for divorce. Over the course of a month, both chose to change and to lean toward strengths. First priority, they decided how to get the work done and balance the salaries in accord with business generation. Second, they prioritized Brenda's job for routine expectations, making sure she used her guru strengths. Stress was lessened; Brenda returned to full workday hours and establishing status quo was possible. Could this relationship be saved sooner? They had to learn before they could earn. Too bad they didn't understand earlier that money means different things to each personality and consciousness precedes action.

Powerbroker Lawyer and Pleasure Seeker Party Planner:

Gina told us that "Steve is almost every girl's dream: popular, good-looking, smart, very rich, sings as good as Elvis, etc, etc." A Pleasure Seeker with money, however, he was nothing like his wife, Gina, a Powerbroker lawyer. Instead of being a big spender, as Gina had believed, he was the biggest saver. How could he behave so opposite of what she expected? Steve planned parties for a living — not little parties, but big parties for congressional candidates. He did not attend those parties or "party" in any other sense of the word, just plan all the details! His family and religious background did not accept dancing and drinking. No drinking, partying and no dancing in this spouse's repertoire. Steve acted like a perfect Problem Solver in everyday life but tested like as Pleasure Seeker. Could he mask his real financial personality?

If something did not change, Gina related that she was doomed to boredom. Being female and a Powerbroker, she had an internal message that says if you love me, you'll want to spend time and attention on me (not save time for the future — spend some now). She comes in Friday night after a hard week at work and is still on the fast track. She wants to go somewhere nice, spend some money, or minimally socialize. She would even be content to let her spouse enjoy his "Elvis music" if they would invite friends over for food, drink, conversation and games. She wanted some input regarding money, weekends and Steve's time.

Being male, Steve equated love with respect. He had been raised in a quiet home that valued music, and he wanted Gina to respect his need for solitude. He'd just as soon lock the door on Friday night after a hard week at work planning parties and not see anyone until Monday. He would squash her suggestions with comments like "You don't need to go there, you don't want to do that." They inherently knew what they personally needed but not what the other needed. How easy it is to forget that "other" means other, different, not the same as you.

Where is a compromise for this story? Statistically speaking, opposites attract, and then have the capability of driving each other crazy for the rest of their lives. This couple had taken their similarities and driven them into opposites. The goal for this couple was to lean toward strengths that originally attracted them. This helped break the impasse. Reminiscing about their initial attraction, it was clear that Steve was more Pleasure Seeker but had adopted family values that helped balance the big spender Gina. Behind closed doors, Steve secretly thought he needed to "fix" Gina. She must be broken to want to spend so much money solely on entertainment — she must not know what was really good for her. Today, they say they work to meet in the middle: Gina feels like Steve recaptured his spirit and he feels like she is maturing, willing to reevaluate their wants and needs around money and time.

CHAPTER ELEVEN

Birds Of A Feather Flock Together
&
How To Make That Work

11

⚮

Young couples today typically haven't heard the expression "Birds of a feather flock together," and often ask for an explanation. For our **Millionaire Code** purpose, it means that people bond and work better together through their shared traits rather than dissimilar leanings.

Most of us can recount experiences with a group of strangers where we are drawn to those we think are "just like us." It is so easy to discuss work, schedules, vacations, hobbies, investments, politics, and even money with people who seem to understand just what we are communicating. Pleasure Seekers often laugh when each guesses what the other is about to say or both are passionate (and loud) about the same subject. Powerbrokers get on the fast tract together and may even leave the gathering to finish their conversation. Problem Solvers express relief at finding someone who is turned off to jokes and interested in what is "really important." Peacemakers are just glad to find someone else to sit down with and watch the comings and goings. It often turns out that all are different in significant ways, but they are bonded more often by likes than dislikes.

For personalities coming together for business or marriage, we recognize that relationships are created because opposites attract *and* birds of a feather enjoy one another's company. While same-personality relationships seem easier before the wedding, many couples find out exactly how different they are in the day-to-day marriage. As a result, this chapter has one main purpose: To show how to break a strangulating **Millionaire Code** "hold" for partners who are just alike. Shared money goals based on a balanced financial plan works wonders. Partners inherently know something about the other's moods and drive. They make a more intelligent and consensual inference about wants and needs. The only problem comes when both partners lean toward *both* of their weaknesses with money at the same time. They compete with each other. And so it's said that two heads are better than one, but not when they're both operating on the same personality flaws. Consider the following double doses of strengths or weaknesses.

1. Pleasure Seeker Partnership

Partners who share Pleasure Seeker traits are loads of fun. They're cheerful, friendly and have a fun-loving outlook. Obviously, having fun together helps them overlook many problems. They are both people magnets and enjoy being with lots of people. They typically know the latest and greatest fads, the best purchases, and strive to own them. This partnership is the *"proverbial Jones"* that others strive to emulate. The only bad news is that they compete for money and for an audience. Entertaining audiences, having ongoing fun, and pleasure seeking, all at the same time, can be expensive. There is always something fun to add to their arsenal of fun things — swimming pools come before new roofs, and cruises before retirement plan contributions, and fun before bills are paid.

If *neither* spouse has any inkling of perfect Problem Solver strengths, there will be no respect for details and budgets. Today looks rosy with checks in their pocket, money in the ATM, or at least credit on the card. However, tomorrow may be a briar patch, a maze of thorns as a result of having so much darn fun. The *somewhat* good news is that neither spouse will fall apart over the problems.

Fix The Obvious Flaws In The Ointment!

You may not have agreed with 100% of the "a" answers on the money personality test, and you didn't have to. You only had to agree with a majority to be primarily a Pleasure Seeker with money. Examine the big picture in the following list of strengths and weaknesses inherent in this personality. Do you see the fly- or the flaw-in-the-ointment?

PLEASURE SEEKER STRENGTHS	PLEASURE SEEKER FLAWS
1. They work to live and live for today. 2. Money buys fun and that's not all there is to happiness but it is valued for good times, and good memories. 3. No one job or disappointment is viewed at cataclysmic for future earnings. 4. When there really is "leftover money," they have the shopping list ready, ... 5. And the competitive pricing to match. 6. They love Monopoly, a great game of strategy that reinforces the assets of real estate investment, profit/loss lessons. 7. They value relationships, creativity, and sharing, service to and with others. 8. Life is an adventure; don't limit it!	1. They don't track accessible/available cash, SO... 2. They spend money they don't have; "leftover" money after bills is often elusive. 3. They can't live in the future SO when it comes to long-term savings, they are angry and stressed 4. The triple D's: dates, details, deadlines — poor memory for each. 5. Monopoly has clear rules but real life fudges on outcomes, e.g., sleep problems, worry, anxious, short fuses. 6. They do have the strongest tendencies among any personality to just spend more than they make, save or invest.

Eight strengths compared to six weaknesses, not a bad ratio. Pleasure Seekers have more financial strengths than weaknesses, but their flaws can be extremely expensive and tip the scale away from unlocking their **Millionaire Code**. All too often trouble starts out as fun. What's our prescription for hanging on to that positive attitude and a long life of fun? Tip the scale back toward strengths with four relatively easy (albeit time intensive) resolutions:

1. Consider your possible need for multiple checking accounts: Two individual accounts and one joint account to pay bills, reserve all important allowances for taxes, quarterly insurance payments, etc. Joint means joint monies — joint access for groceries and other housing bills. If one has a gripe about grocery bills, both should go to the store until price shock wears off. If one doesn't like the heating bills, try conserving and layering clothing. If you continue to do what you have always done, you will continue to get what you always got — a short fuse, easily distracted, sleeplessness, and worry. These outcomes are in direct opposition to unlocking your **Millionaire Codes** and, in fact, could break the freewheeling spirit. Individual accounts could be for individual responsibilities or for each to use as their own "leftover" money that can be carried over to the next month for a significant purchase or spent on the purchase du jour.

2. Instead of saving for a rainy day, save for a sunny day. Buckle down with a calendar and a financial plan to secure your nest egg. According to the millionaires we've researched, they put away anywhere from 10% to 25% in separate savings accounts just for incidentals, car breakdowns, a new car, household appliances, medicines, etc.

3. Interview and price the plans for three different Certified Financial Planners (CFPs) before hiring someone who will challenge, not over power, your personality. They can help analyze your nest egg needs according to your age and stage in life. But educate yourself financially and don't pawn off all responsibilities on any professional.

4. Reevaluate insurance for health, life, housing, and cars. Do not confuse insurance with investments.

Time consuming, yes, but these four steps can address costly flaws and let you get back to more love and more fun, leaning toward financial strengths.

2. The Powerbroker Partnership

A marriage between spouses that share Powerbroker traits is rich and action packed. Each carries the subconscious mental checklists common to powerful personalities. They gleefully busy themselves with accomplishing more tasks than seems humanly possible. Their drive and lifestyle are often dizzying to their family and friends. The good news is that each is also amazed with the other's task orientation and appreciative of accomplishments (+$$$). The bad news is that they unconsciously compete with each other to see who can accomplish the "most" goals; and without steadily investing in savings, successful goal completion can cost big bucks (-$$$). Neither is good at watching the pot of gold; they are too busy putting it to work and polishing it so they can see their own reflection.

For these guys, vacations are for seeing and doing new things, not for resting. They may even combine business with pleasure, and both are happy with that. They have dreams, established goals, accomplished dreams and continually create more dreams followed by more goals. Dollar watching is expected and accomplished. Deadlines are expected and accomplished. Oh, sure, they can have problems. They might lean toward weaknesses to resolve who is the most right at any one point in time, but they quickly find areas for agreement. Forgiveness of infractions is possible but forgetting the infraction rarely happens. Each has the memory that never forgets!

Remember To Use Your Strengths

This couple does not mince words, so we won't either. Hopefully, one or both have blended personalities so they can examine their strengths and weaknesses and look at the big picture.

PERSONALITY STRENGTHS FOR POWERBROKER RELATIONSHIPS	PERSONALITY FLAWS FOR POWERBROKER RELATIONSHIPS
1. Work consistently fast, hard, and dedicated, e.g., usually long hours. 2. Builds up good credit records. 3. Keeps money in motion, working for them. 4. Understands what makes them happy, money, power, self-control. 5. Good with numbers, making big plans and specific goals. 6. Future oriented with financial plans. 7. Expects investments to perform. 8. Watches/tracks financial performance. 9. Competitive shoppers. 10. Make good decisions about money. 11. Takes charge, control of finances. 12. It is personally challenging and invigorating to make more money. 13. Will get their financial plan done!	1. Workaholic. 2. Thinks credit is the best invention and only tracks win-win earnings. 3. Money moves too fast and they don't foresee the long-term impact. 4. No money? The outcome is no self-confidence, power, or self-control. 5. The big picture is visible, but the details are invisible. 6. The future comes in six months. Long-term is futuristic. If investment doesn't perform, ditch it; move on (too fast). 7. Big spender. 8. Distrusts negative but realistic facts! 9. Expects to control everybody's destiny. 10. High levels of competition make them more headstrong, critical (ulcerous). 11. Wants to plan then spend their way.

Thirteen strengths and eleven potential traps put strengths ahead, but only *if* both partners recognize the problems in time to put on a positive spin. The personality flaws are as strongly negative as the strengths are passionately positive. Any one of the eleven flaws can be a significant setback to unlocking their **Millionaire Code**, more like breaking the bank. Imagine two people on the fast track in the Olympics who are supposed to pass off to each other in the relay but end up racing each other to the finish line. It's definitely not a win-win situation, but a lot of times this couple may not care. It is not hard for these people to break into **The Millionaire Code**; the tough part comes in trying to keep it. Consider the following prescription for unlocking then leaning into your **Millionaire Code**.

1. You want money for power and control, and a lot of people are glad for you to make the money and take the helm. However, practice self-control not over-powering others, particularly your partner, because they will take it as a challenge and compete with you for like purposes.

2. Spend less than you earn on lifestyle.

3. Pay off high-interest credit cards within the expected time frame.

4. Don't borrow to invest in the stock or bond market.

5. Realize that your strength in understanding numbers, graphs and charts over months with an eye toward "the future" is sharp. However, your passion tends to fall short of any realistic definition of "long-term." If you live within your means but don't have extended "long-term" savings and investments, you may be "average" (and we know you hate that) — in and out of the 3.5 Club many times over. Average is not your style.

6. Search out objective sources for investments, financial plans, insurance and secure a nest egg. Buy, but don't get sold down the river because you are in a hurry to get back on the fast track.

3. Problem Solver Partnership

Partners who share the perfect problem-solver traits are typically the picture of success. They consider themselves equally well educated, value a nice home (not too fancy) and safe, long-lasting cars (not necessarily fun or fast, but *just* right). Long-term means what it should — years into the future. They have retirement funds, planned vacations, and the future is planned to stay on target. They enjoy family time as well as a nice balance of time with a small, close circle of friends. They are typically faithful, respectful and devoted. They tend to be generous with what they have, including time and possessions. They listen to each other's complaints because there lies their life's mission: solving problems. They persistently debate and work to solve each other's problems. They are content to stay in the background for one another. Their vacations alternate between action, sometimes even daring or exotic excursions, and restful elopements. Music, art, food and other aesthetic interests are relaxing for both and highly valued.

But, as is true of all human nature, Problem Solvers will fall prey to personality flaws sometime, sooner rather than later, particularly if they don't know what to watch out for. One or both might lean toward their perfectionist weaknesses and set off jointly demonstrated negative attitudes, suspicion, alienation, pessimism and very hard to please behaviors. All flaws have costs. The ill-gotten chain of reactions can be easily broken using shared traits such as overly analytical, self-sacrificing, considerate, and respectful.

So, Problem Solver, Why Aren't You Perfect Yet?

No one is perfect, but you are complete with all the traits you need to unlock **The Millionaire Code**.

However, you are only human. Family dollars somehow take on a life of their own, and you try to work for them. It is supposed to be the other way around — your dollars are supposed to work for you. You are such a good planner and so conscientious about everything, you can't fathom how finances can somehow, sometimes get out of control. You are the sequential Problem Solver, and money can be a problem, but rarely a permanent problem for the "thinker," which you are. While you will no doubt deny that you are emotional, one-fourth of human beings are perfect Problem Solvers, and their traits include more "moodiness," more emo-

PROBLEM SOLVER STRENGTHS	PROBLEM SOLVER FLAWS
1. Balance and organize time for both work and play.	1. You procrastinate. While your intention is flawless and your plan for handling the family finances is good, it taxes you to start (& you put it off too long) because you don't want to do it unless you do it *right!*
2. Know how much money is saved, needed for expenses and accessible for lifestyle.	
3. Save for rainy days and retirement.	
4. Value $ for security, clear conscious.	
5. Live and spend within means.	2. Perfectionist financial analysts are not exempt from flaw #1 because they "do it" all day & don't want to come home for more of the same.
6. Left over money preferably is saved.	
7. Design detailed budgets.	
8. Most purchases are a result of thinking and organizing.	3. Learning about investments and insurance always sounds like a scam. You get what you pay for & this goes for the very security you value.
9. Shop brand names, look for sales.	
10. Monthly money management is a thoughtful process.	4. You can't decide; you return more than you keep and can be stressed in a state of need (often for basics, like in #3).
11. Watch details, analyze, calculate choices.	
12. Very sensitive about other's financial problems and needs. Tries to be generous.	5. Financial stress is overwhelming & often influences sleeping and eating, moods, ability to remedy the problem.

tional sensitivities about a lot of issues. You have so many strengths; don't deny your weaknesses. Consider the following prescription for unlocking your **Millionaire Code**.

1. Don't love your money; it won't love you back.

2. If you are not a financial analyst, get busy and educate yourself about the big picture involved in financial planning. Getting wrapped up in the details is good, but it may not get you where you want or need to be. Don't let details become burdens.

3. You want money for security and a clear conscience. Fine! Some security can be bought through proper levels and different types of health, home, life and car insurance, as well as umbrella policies. Since you don't like to talk to these folks, books, brochures and internet disclosures are probably your best avenue for getting accurate information. But trust somebody sometime!

4. Self-insure! More security can be had with money market funds, certificates of deposits, or I-BONDS that rise with inflation and can't fall with deflation (www.savingsbonds.gov). Keeping some money on the sidelines, boring and safe, is good. But when the *basics* are *basically* handled, address the big picture issue with inflation more seriously.

5. Secure your nest egg. Invest steadily by putting whatever you can comfortably afford into one or two "index funds" or no-load, low-expense stock market mutual funds.

6. When you first feel guilty about dropping one of the many balls you constantly have in the air, identify it as a problem, lean toward your problem solving strengths and make your weaknesses the fly in the ointment.

4. The Peacemaker Partnership

The Peacemaker household is a very comfortable home. Their mantra is to keep it easy, relaxed, and consistently peaceful. Serenity and price conscious comforts are priorities. As far as the Peacemaker is concerned, cheap is chic. In good times and in bad, under pressure and stress, both parties look for the easy way; neither is trying to light a fire under the other. Neither is easily moved to action, on anything. They are pleasant and enjoyable, good listeners, with many friends. They talk on a need to know basis and are happy living on the couch.

The Peacemaker personality comes out dead even, 50% strengths and 50% weaknesses. What will tip the scale and turn "Home Sweet Home" into "Home Sour Home?" The propensity to be a couch potato and do nothing! While lying around is great in the comfort of home, it is not so nice in relationships when one partner needs more. For example, it might be that one needs a nice new couch, but, seriously, it might be more personal. Two Peacemakers in partnership don't always see eye-to-eye, and they have a difficult time communicating. When they do bring up any concern, *anything* can seem like a problem, new responsibilities, the opposite of peace at any price.

The real message behind "peace at any price" is "avoid conflict." Maybe the two partners inherently know this but don't know how to avoid conflict when there is an issue at hand. The Peacemaker typically responds with behavior that is intended to intimidate the other person into not bringing up the issue — a passive look, the look that would kill, or a nonchalant "let's see." To avoid conflict, understand your weaknesses, talk more and consider the following to uncover your **Millionaire Code**.

1. The Peacemaker has so many strengths with money: competent and steady, peaceful with administrative capability, *mediates* problems, finds the easy way. Watching money, which is their preference, is not enough!

2. When you allow yourself to honestly think that failure is an option, what you are really doing is trying to challenge your partner to do something you are not willing to do — take action. You want to put all of the responsibility on someone else, but your behavior is showing. You are admitting that your laziness is a problem.

3. Doubt is inherent *only* when you lean toward your weaknesses. You doubt yourself, others, and almost any definitive action. Your "policies" sound so consistent like peace at any price, we'll get around to it, slow and steady wins the race, but they can be excuses for inaction.

PEACEMAKER STRENGTHS	PEACEMAKER FLAWS
1. Time and money have a direct correlation: slow and steady wins the race.	1. There is still "a race," a human race, meaning that like it or not, the value of goods and services often moves faster than you wish (e.g., both up and down).
2. Money is a personal subject.	
3. Stashes incoming money in safe havens and forget about it.	2. Your money behavior is showing.
4. Money means self-respect and a certain status in the family of well being.	3. Stashes incoming money in safe havens (good) and *forget about it* (not so good).
5. It is important to financially help family in trouble.	4. We hear Peacemakers say, "Failure is always an option (with money)," but is it?
6. Left over money is immediately saved.	5. What is the most common problem in loans to family? They resent it as a loan — there is a need to clarify loan or gift, or be resented!
7. Waits and watches approach to handling money, particularly savings.	
8. Watches what others buy, discern the value and then decide if it's good for me/us.	6. May be the guru, but hoarding money, not asking your spouse about unmet needs makes you a jerk.
9. Specialty stores limit choices in goods for quality purchases; they are right for me.	7. Wait & watch does not guarantee good investment or peace of mind.
10. Monthly money management? Deposit it and forget it!	8. Watches others because you doubt yourself.
	9. Peace at any price? Not consistently practiced; real policy is "avoid conflict."
	10. Financial planning? I'll get round to it.

4. While outsiders looking in may see stability, you know the truth. Don't deny personality flaws. Watch for instability from inactivity.

In summary, breaking **The Millionaire Code** requires knowing your personality traits, leaning toward strengths, seeking to understand, and encouraging the multiple strengths of others. If only one partner understands the personal and relationship needs of others, amazing changes take place. New thoughts can create new responses. Behavior changes more easily when people get what they need and are unconditionally loved for who they are instead of who *you* want them to be.

Millionaire Code Stories

TRUE STORY — For the Fun of It

Julie and Steve were just alike, both Pleasure Seekers and newlyweds!

They competed — for spending money, time, attention, and for respect of each person's need to spend time, attention AND money with separate sets of friends.

Then, they saw the light (or the darkness) at the end of "fun" and decided to follow the financial personality guidelines. They set up a meeting with a certified financial planner. The new couple wanted to make sure that they established their financial plan so that they could get energized about their future together. Steve completed the financial forms as requested and the financial analyst examined the information. In an attempt to ascertain their attitude about money, the analyst asked the young couple a series of questions regarding their financial history and spending habits.

Their current financial picture spelled disaster, two big cars with loans and leases, jewelry, vacation timeshares, cruises, no assets like a house. You name it — everything pointed to financial ruin. They were both big, really big spenders. They had been spending for years before they were married, and both were spending more now than they made. Should they hang it up, split up or file for bankruptcy?

Of course not — marriages between like personalities are not a death sentence with no chance of parole! Will success involve change? Absolutely. They will need to adopt their **Millionaire Code** strengths and subsequently change their spending and shopping behavior. The two of them make good income. They can immediately address the disproportionate huge outlay of cash monthly for two financed cars and try to sell or quit investing in worthless timeshares. They will need to defer their dreams of executive reservations on cruises. They need a new dream about investments (maybe a home or other tax shelter). They will need to change the way they spend and save joint money and develop a financial plan, essential for two Pleasure Seekers. Communication about money wants and needs must become habit, at least every paycheck, and definitely not over a glass of wine (which is their temptation — let's have fun!).

Too much peace is no good.

An especially peaceful, laid back couple joined our educational seminar for "no specific reason." They had come simply to see if they could learn to "peaceably" work together on issues that involved money. On what issues did they need to work? With peaceful smiles on their faces, they admitted they were deadlocked. Mary said she wanted a different house, newer, more fitting for their empty nest status. Bob said, "It costs too much." Mary retorted, "Everything costs too much." Bob had been saving forever and had plenty of money. Mary had her own money. But he was even negative and pessimistic about her spending her money.

Then she relayed the real reasons why she wanted a different house. It cost too much to fix the bathroom sink that had needed repair for a year. Last week the sink ripped away from the wall. Now Bob is convinced it costs too much to fix the sink and the wall. "Use the kitchen sink," he says. But Jean told us that the kitchen sink was antiquated and rusty. However, she didn't want to complain because the buckets Bob used for repairs reliably caught drips from around the caulk. The appliances were untrustworthy. She could not get a burner to turn off, so now it was disconnected.

The finale came when she described the room that had been added years ago to the back of the house. A tree had fallen on the roof last winter and it was still there, six months later. It costs too much to remove it! If that wasn't enough, Jean quietly and demurely told us that it was especially confusing why her husband would financially bail out their "deadbeat" college-age kids but not allow her to make their home "comfortable." Bob was definitely hard to motivate and resented being pushed.

Bob needed a dose of logical consequences, so instead of

pushing, we pulled him into the real world. He could look forward to either his or his wife's physical and mental disorders from various states of ill repair ($$$). Or maybe the whole house falling or burning down would wake him up ($$$). Try no resale value (-$$$) until repairs are made (for someone else to enjoy) or the inability to sell house (-$$$). Being inherently concerned about what others think, maybe it would bother him to face litigious complaints from neighbors. And, of course, there is always his inability to cover costs of living while money is buried under the mattress (-$$$). Then there is the lack of respect (status) he was encouraging from his wife and kids (priceless). Last but not least, he was insuring no possible peace of mind. The costs, as a result of his locking up his **Millionaire Code** were huge. He's now "thinking" about it. Maybe he'll get around to it.

Healthy, Wealthy And Wise: When To Listen To The Strengths—Not The Weaknesses

12
∞

Once upon a time, in the 1950s to be exact, there was a revered money trick — one guaranteed to reduce stress and worry. This practice, known to most psychiatrists and psychologists of the time, foreshadowed the scientific link between money and mental health. Amazingly, this common sense technique remained in wide practice even as mental health was "waking up" to more and more scientific strategies. While insulin and electro-convulsive shock, major and minor tranquilizers, and hospitalizations ruled the day, many a professional imparted this one cheap psychological trick to their patients.

And so the white-coated professional would say to his patient: "If you want to feel better, take a $100 bill and keep it in your wallet or purse at all times. Don't spend it, just keep it there." Put another way: "There's no drug that works as well as a roll of money hidden in your wallet or bank drawer." In other words, if you have money, you may have worries, and granted money doesn't buy happiness, but money — a $100 bill — can go a long way towards reducing stress and worry. It doesn't stop the pain, but it does provide a kind of mental secret weapon that promotes confidence and reduces stress.

In today's society, the credit card has largely replaced the confidence of having that $100 bill, but it's not the same thing. In fact, using a credit card will achieve the opposite effect. With no money and only bills, that brief sense of feeling good is now replaced with the reality of limited cash. Stress and worries are exacerbated; a vicious cycle kicks in; and that's the point. Money impacts your health status, and that's why we've chosen this as our final chapter. In good health and in bad, how you handle money and concomitant debts can affect you both physical and mentally. It's impossible to face the world, to swim effectively upstream, and to counteract the "slings and arrows of outrageous fortune" when we are persistently tired, sick or injured. It's even harder when there's no money to fight with.

As a result, it's time you understood how your "financial personality" and your "fitness personality" work together to unlock your **Millionaire Code.** Simply put, you can't spend money on fun, power, security, or peace of mind if you're not healthy. And if you don't understand this relationship, someone else (your health professionals) will have the privilege of spending your hard-earned cash. To explain this link between money and health, here's a look at what people hate most: exercise.

Newsweek polled 1,200 people about their exercise dollars, numbers and attitude (DNA!). Ninety-three per cent said they believe exercise is critical to good physical health. However, only 63% walk around the block at least three times per week (even *Newsweek* didn't think that was sufficient for good health). A small percentage of respondents did more but the rest did less than little to nothing.

This is no surprise. Most people unconsciously play to their personality weaknesses. They're like old friends, familiar and comforting — even though they cause problems. The excuses not to exercise fit their financial personality. See for yourself.

Why don't you exercise?	Male	Female	Personality
I don't have time!	53%	36%	Powerbrokers
I hate it I know I'm lazy	9%	19%	Peacemakers
I'm okay — I already have active lifestyle	11%	12%	Pleasure Seekers
I feel *fine*; I don't care about it	10%	10%	Problem Solvers
No answer	17%	23%	Your guess?

To further demonstrate how your financial personality and your fitness personality are related, we did a six-month study at a posh Atlanta country club. Here's what we found.

Pleasure Seeker's Health

Pleasure Seekers are naturally breezy, friendly, spontaneous and enthusiastic if they stay fit. Off kilter, however, people pleasers can become distracted, flighty, and exhibit a bundle of free-floating anxiety. This is not good for tennis teams and each member needs to support the physical health of others. Once this personality is off-physical balance, they worry more, sleep less, and have a short fuse that easily ignites. Many a temper tantrum has been witnessed at sports events, little league games and tennis courts. Obviously this can cost relationships, but lately the news has shocked us with resulting lawsuits over wrongful deaths from such explosive behaviors. Once lawyers get involved, unlocking those **Millionaire Codes** will be put on hold for years.

Since Pleasure Seekers tend to get their energy in fits and starts, bursts and spurts, they push their bodies to the limit and then crash. These individuals respond best to exercise that calms their chattering thoughts, uses space creatively, and stretches and balances them. Typically they need to exercise with a workout buddy, one that allows them to sweat and to socialize simultaneously. While all personalities will play tennis, Pleasure Seekers tend to sign up in significant numbers, and this is a good *popular* activity. Unfortunately, they may be unreliable players, physically and emotionally, habitually late for the warm up and totally ignore the need for toning and building muscle. Because the bursts and spurts leave them with injuries that tax their **Millionaire Code**, tennis may not be the only exercise they need. They need to think outside the tennis court.

To get them to do more, we would appeal to their strengths. They would savor the chance to talk and walk fast for 45 minutes straight or participate with a congenial group lifting weights, dancing, or doing yoga. But will they do it? Will they use their

Millionaire Code? Chances are, "they will be too busy."

Powerbroker's Health

The Powerbroker has the discipline to excel at fitness. When in balance, they smolder with passions and WOW everyone with knowledge about the challenge of sport. Out of balance, however, they scorch others (and their checkbooks) with unreasonable demands, criticism, confrontation and long-lasting injuries. Their healthy desire for challenge turns into a fixation on winning. Winning "what?" is exactly "what" needs to be reevaluated. Stress mounts with increasing impatience in traffic, in lines, *even* for a machine at the gym (hence the reminders for people to get off the machines at exactly 45 minutes). Their no-nonsense approach to exercise is to get in, get going and get out. The best workout is a hard workout. Unfortunately, this often leads to significant injuries ($$$), even burnout. This personality naturally succeeds in both money matters and health matters. However, they must take the focus off "winning" when it comes to fitness and put it on self-control and individual power. Disciplined exercise, martial arts, yoga, hiking, biking, skiing and rowing can provide needed balance. Set goals and record progress!

Problem Solver's Health

In balance, Problem Solvers can be calm, cool, geniuses with money and relationships as well as curious explorers. Out of balance, they look for perfection in all the wrong places. They overeat or starve, oversleep, exhibit moodiness and suffer through digestive problems, stomachaches, spleen and liver imbalances, even muscle and joint pain. Once they decide to move onto something, they have super strength and endurance. When it comes to exercise, they thrive on change.

They enjoy alternating kickboxing with aerobics, adventure weekends with circuit training classes, and finally, outdoor runs interspersed with rock climbing. They do them all perfectly. They prefer twosomes or small, close-knit groups for trekking across the globe, but can also easily adjust to videotape, early morning TV programs or small-group instruction. They need to remember that perfect performance is decidedly elusive. Leaning toward their weaknesses, they will quit everything for weeks on end! This is not conducive to health or money management! To get them back on track they should be encouraged to do what they enjoy and build on past successful experiences.

Peacemaker's Health

The Peacemaker has a slow metabolism and their demeanors are more laid back, even laid down. They thrive on relaxation but can easily lapse into procrastination. When unbalanced, they can have symptoms of congestion, sinus, lung, kidney problems, asthma and lethargy. They are the embodiment of the modern couch potato. Being big music or TV fans, they (honestly) can get great exercise by taking their audio players on the road and hike, bike, or even watch TV on a treadmill, stepper or in a recumbent bike (it reclines!). Setting small goals like training for a half-K marathon (no exaggeration intended) and keeping track of progress can be a strong motivator for the Peacemaker's good health and strong wealth.

Three-Sided Sword

Fitness is a two-sided dagger — physical and mental — throw in money, and it's a three-sided sword. The relationship between physical fitness and emotional/mental fitness goes at least two ways — physical problems have emotional consequences, and emotional problems have physical consequences. Each complicates money, *but* each personality comes complete with all the strengths needed for *mental fitness*.

Unfortunately, into every life some stress will fall. While stress is today's buzzword for physical and mental symptoms, it's actually the body's "nonspecific" response to any demand placed on it, either real or imagined. Nonspecific simply implies that the responses are individualized, by personality and by personal history, age and stage of life. Any stress, *good* or bad, causes a physiological response in your body producing chemicals that prepare men for fight or flight and women for befriending. The trick is to keep it from running wild and avoiding overload.

When that happens, anyone can experience anxiety, withdrawal, physical illness, even rage, and fall into traps involving violence, promiscuity, drug addiction and bankruptcy. Fortunately, there's a remedy, if you choose it. Recognize your personality stress style. Problem solving and stress responses are not always the same, so here's a strategy for each financial personality.

Peacemaker Mental Fitness

Try to understand and eliminate stress by using friends and family for support. Unfortunately, you often withdraw and cut off communication, and then make poor decisions in a vacuum. The Peacemaker's need for peace and consistent order, when taken to the extreme, results in fearful doubting, procrastination, bullying with silence and a lack of decisiveness. There is no situation that we can think of today that has less predictability and order than financial status and wealth management. Enter stress! Enter procrastination and indecisiveness! Enter lethargy, breathing problems, congestion and annoying allergies, and other truly "in your face" physical pains, all a direct affront and assault to peace of mind. It is a vicious circle.

Recommendation: Your strength is to be proactive, and your weakness is to be reactive. You want the easiest way to get back to the status quo, but the good in status quo is often elusive. Staying calm, cool and collected in times of trouble is key. Check your fitness status and schedule exercise. Reflect on the bigger picture surrounding the problem instead of on the specific stress. Talk with others about possible choices to resolve the problem. Finding a peaceful solution is good; being lazy and procrastinating will cost you time and money.

Powerbroker Mental Fitness

When you have a problem, you focus on a solution and don't

let others get in the way. Sometimes, however, in looking for the fast way, you miss the real problem and face more hurt than help. Powerbrokers need a certain degree of independence and productivity. When taken to extremes, they easily lose track and flip over to domineering, demanding, and workaholic behaviors. Their sensitivity to competitive challenges by others may even result in vengeful rage. Money is so important to them that money stress and lack of control over money can cause them even bigger problems like heartburn, stomach ulcers.

Recommendation: Slow down and try to make notes about the problem from a couple of viewpoints. Set goals, physical, mental and situation specific and create win-win scenarios. Don't be so quick to compete — recognize that there's value in cooperation. Not every challenge should be treated as an emergency that needs a fast decision. It's possible to be a leader and cooperate at the same time. While this may not suit your ego, it's time you learned that anyone can be a success if they don't mind who gets the credit.

Pleasure Seeker Mental Fitness

You nurture and comfort others and readily share, but ignore your own stressful problems. Sometimes you try and wash them away with fun times — even fun drinks. And, of course, there's shopping, certainly a potentially expensive therapy. Each of these reactions serves to temporarily whitewash the problem; but, as you well know, the problem comes back, stronger than ever, and packed with a vengeance. It's not solved; it's just back, and the physical components of these problems never went away.

Recommendation: First, find a personal way to calm the chattering mind. Check your health and fitness status. Then prioritize the issues involved in your problem, just as you would help others do. Decide which elements are in your control and which ones are not. Address the ones in your control first. Identify pros, cons *and* your feelings about each of at least two solutions, then listen to others' feedback (we know you will request that!), summarize the big picture and ask for help getting the job done just right.

Problem Solver Mental Fitness

How can the Problem Solver ignore problems? Simple, one problem is challenging; but two or more, particularly ones that are interrelated, retard and physically depress the problem solving machinery. Deadlines are particularly upsetting, and money management is laden with frustrating deadlines. You plan and plan, and plan some more to solve problems, and in the process of planning, set standards that are untimely, often too high and out of reach. The Problem Solver needs purpose and wants to help others. When taken to the extreme, these sensitivities cause them to get depressed, pessimistic, judgmental and unforgiving. They want perfection. When taken to extreme, they will withdraw completely or become revengeful. Digestive, muscle and joint pains are common and even troublesome to diagnose.

Recommendation: Check you diet and fitness status since both plummet when under stress. Strive to be less judgmental with others when you are under stress; and, if you can, give yourself permission to be less judgmental of yourself. Once you quit beating yourself up, reevaluate your definition of security. True security comes from self-confidence. Be true to your value system, then get back to the task at hand which is to creatively find solutions, a very valuable strength!

In summary, any personality can think negatively during times of high stress and allow their financial personality to foment money mistakes. The Pleasure Seekers will conclude there is no fun to be had, grow distracted from priorities, and radiate worry and free-floating anxiety. The Powerbrokers will conclude that they have lost control and lose their cool to fiery passion; they tend to fall back on win-lose strategies (they win, you lose!). The Problem Solvers will determine that things are not going right; their ordinary proactive stance becomes a reactive response, depressing them and others around them. The Peacemaker will feel disengaged when there is no peace in sight. They tend to go blank, meaning they quit trying to understand or to mediate, and they become aimless, doubtful, indecisive, and then (the financial nightmare) indifferent.

There's no way to completely eliminate stress; in fact, it can help us perform better. It is common sense and proven psychology that better stress management is a preventive approach: know who you are, who you were meant to be, and play up your strengths. The Pleasure Seeker wants control to do things the *fun* way but needs to habitually keep priorities straight. The Powerbroker wants control to do things *their* way but must balance this drive and competitiveness with win-win strategies. The Problem Solver wants control to do things the *right* way but needs to analyze reactive behavior that is the opposite of their proactive modus operandi. The Peacemaker wants control to do things the *easy* way but will have to struggle to avoid habitual procrastination and to squash doubt.

How can you decide where to invest your energies? How can you evaluate what stresses possibly deserve less attention, less focus in your everyday activities? Each financial personality is motivated to avoid pain and enjoy pleasure by their personal definition. Some are more motivated by pain avoidance and some are more motivated with seeking pleasure. Observing and understanding your DNA, your behavior surrounding dollars, numbers and attitude is essential.

But "understanding" is not the end goal; behavior change and self-control is the hallmark of de-stress success. We can and will feel stress in the 22nd century. However, as soon as we decide (purposefully) that a situation is no longer cataclysmic, dangerous and stressful, we can take the necessary steps to change our monetary wants and needs — our **Millionaire Code**. Few situations have no solutions, so as soon as we focus on what we are good at, rapid changes can occur in our minds and bodies to help us relax and approach money difficulties and problems methodically.

Financial De-Stress

How can you purposely tell your brain to slow down the adrenaline rush that naturally occurs when you sense financial stress, whether it be good or bad? The same mechanism that turns the stress response on can turn it off! The opposite of the stress inducing sympathetic nervous system is the parasympathetic nervous system — responsible for rest, relaxation, food digestion, injury repair, growth, the immune system and all of the body's essential housekeeping chores. The relaxation response includes decreased heart and breathing rate, sense of well being, and peace. Adults who develop a personal 'relaxation response' feel less helpless and have more choices when responding to stress. Stress management is not a "natural ability;" you have to learn it and cultivate it. Here are some techniques to help you do just that.

The four primary relaxation exercises (in contrast to *energizing* exercises) are deep breathing, journaling, mental rehearsal and imagery awareness. All four personalities benefit from learning these techniques; but as you can guess, there's one technique that works best for each personality. They work because your **Millionaire Code** benefits from physically energizing exercise and relaxation exercises.

Too much of a good thing like energizing usually needs to be balanced with relaxation. For example, the Pleasure Seeker enjoys friendships, conversation and is sensitive to rejection. Being a creative storyteller, they "journal" naturally — witness their scribbling throughout meetings when they are not the speakers. Expand the idea to journal feelings through writing about negative, unwanted feelings of rejection. It is OKAY to acknowledge negative feelings if you know you are trying to get back to positive feelings. Those negative feelings tend to gain a new perspective when they are written down on paper (it is easier to see where to start if you know how you want things to end!). Rejection which is inevitable some time, some place, brings anxiety that tends to precipitate shallow breathing. Therefore learning a relaxation response related to "deep breathing" also makes sense.

The Peacemaker, with their tendencies toward congestion and other physical stresses, might also benefit by turning to deep, rhythmic breathing techniques but add imagery awareness. Imagery awareness includes taking a few moments in welcomed silence to visualize being in favorite peaceful locations, be it the beach or mountains (it won't be the hustle and bustle of a city for Peacemakers!). Allow natural breathing to bring visualization for peace of mind. While true peace of mind comes only when your behavior is in harmony with your personality, your principals and your values, visualization of what that entails can be the relaxing first step. The trick for Peacemakers is coming out of that restful state so they will return to mediate problems instead of just watching them stalemate or even grow.

The Problem Solver is a natural daydreamer, so mental rehearsal is their inherent relaxation response and they should capitalize on the technique for relaxation. Mental rehearsal involves visualizing each minute step involved in solving a problem, usually in reverse order (end to beginning). Almost all world-class athletes are visualizers. They see the end result, feel it, and experience it before they ever do it. For example, you may visualize winning a competition or finishing a highly valued product, a painting or song, learning an instrument (or maybe a perfectly balanced financial portfolio? That may be the ultimate challenge in today's economy). The purpose is to start out with the end product in mind and work your way backward, step by small step, visualizing how to go from the end back to the beginning, where you are now with a simple problem.

Journaling is the first line of defense for Powerbrokers because they naturally take notes and outline solutions. However, their normally fast-paced mental checklist needs to be converted to relaxation. This requires a purposeful shift from making one mental checklist to exploring goals from the standpoint of multiple solutions and passions on comparative checklists. The goal is to get away from having only two alternatives — your way and the *wrong* way.

Food For Thought On Personality, Stress, Risk And Reward

What is the relationship between risk tolerance with investments and personality strengths and weaknesses? A person's discomfort or reaction to fluctuations in principal — not interest — determines risk tolerance. A person's response to risk varies over time and over situational experiences. Risk tolerance is variable, an emotional stress quotient, whereas personality is more of a frame for mindfulness. Personality encompasses lifestyle, mood, drive, levels of energy, extroversion or introversion, overall mood, and inherent optimism or realism.

Financial personality codes can be expected to improve or change slightly with age, maturity and health status. We have plenty of strengths (and weaknesses) that are not utilized every season of our lives. Stress happens. Additionally, childhood experiences with poverty or riches can impact financial personality; both leave their mark on emotional IQ and money personality. Extensive losses in personal or family income, including extended bear markets, are like wind shears on emotional stamina, which contributes to risk intolerance. Strengths are always there; but sometimes, they are hard to locate through fog or wind.

However, research shows that personality traits, both strengths and weaknesses, are reliable and stable as much as 66% of the time over any extended period of time. Certainly, one aberrant day, anyone of the four personalities could wake up and decide the markets were right and decide to "risk all." But, given a more thoughtful, extended time period, we tend to revert to inherent personality traits. While introverted personalities are naturally less risk tolerant, they can get caught up in a strong bull market like the extroverted personalities. And even the riskiest Powerbrokers have shut down their tolerance for risk after two years of losing money in a bear market.

In the end, common sense has it that the extroverted personalities of Pleasure Seeker and Powerbroker are naturally more risk tolerant. They are more likely to tolerate larger fluctuations and even loss of principal for the opportunity to reap a higher return. If they lose, their mindset is that they can go back to work tomorrow. Introverted personalities such as Problem Solvers and Peacemakers will be naturally less risk tolerant. Any change in principal causes them concern and a decline of 10% in investments would be grounds for instant retreat. In the end, however, the numbers indicate that personality traits are more stable while risk tolerance is variable.

Millionaire Code Stories

Invest Your Emotions Wisely!

The meeting was typical, one out of 52 during the year designed to resolve routine process-oriented problems among 10 different staff members. All four personalities were around the table. The leader was an extroverted Pleasure Seeker. Staff members were Powerbrokers and perfect Problem Solvers and, lucky for this group, the secretary was a Peacemaker. The leader saw his goal as presenting the big picture. The Problem Solvers are listening for the details and interrupt to contribute. They don't rush through problems. The Powerbrokers rush to solutions since they are on the fast track to get back to work. They act bored with all the input from Problem Solvers. The Peacemaker wants to resolve complaints but gets overwhelmed and nods off (with eyes open). Stress is building.

As soon as the leader listed a third problem, the Problem Solver showed an emotional side, the same one that affects stress levels as well as financial stability. The dynamic goes like this...First someone buries their head in their hands. Then others shake their heads and roll their eyes, silently saying, "oh, no, too much." Others in the room misinterpret the emotional angst, and the Powerbrokers rush in with an all out gripe session. Their behavior was showing. This has happened too many times. The question is, "Can this work relationship be saved?"

Group processes must take into consideration the personalities around the table. The pleasure-seeking leader just wanted to get on with the meeting and was willing to decide issues based on feelings. But so many feelings were nonverbal as well as verbally expressed. The facts are the facts for Powerbrokers, and the details are the details for Problem Solvers. The ineffective group process made the Pleasure Seeker feel easily distracted and worried that no one was happy with their job. Being happy 40+ hours per week was important. He reported sleeping less and being on a short fuse.

Weekly meetings dragged on. The Powerbrokers gossiped critically and grew more headstrong. They had solutions where solutions were not needed. They were not listening. They were popping heartburn medications. The extroverts (Powerbrokers and Pleasure Seekers) were chomping on their pencils. The introverts (Problem Solvers and Peacemakers) became overwhelmed when they were required to go on to the next problem — something they don't like to do unless they feel right with the problem currently on their plate.

The Problem Solvers were meticulous but they over-analyzed details. They do not want to let any issue rest. They prefer to "sort of feel" their way along very slowly and if something doesn't feel right, they "go back to the last place" where they knew they were right and start over again. The Problem Solvers' stresses were leading to burn out. A few were late to work many mornings, reporting fretful sleep then over sleeping. They were generally upset, withdrawn and remote, critical, unforgiving, and frustrated about the job. They appeared to set standards too high (they were failures if unforeseen difficulties cramped their style), were judgmental, suspicious, depressed over imperfections and wallowing in over analysis. They were also "sick" a lot with colds, indigestion, muscle pains and stomach problems.

All of these professionals were very stressed on the job because they did not prioritize where to invest their emotions and all had plenty of emotions. A Gallup Poll of with 1,000,000 participants showed that only 20% of employees use their strengths at work (Buckingham & Clifton, Gallupjournal.com, 2001). What worked? They got educated about personality and group process. Staff members now turn in agenda items the day before routine meetings; the Peacemaker sees how many issues can be resolved before the meeting and presents resolutions as a part of her report. Problem Solvers feel good when the meeting starts with resolved issues. The Pleasure Seeker allows for discussion but respects Powerbroker time limits. They agree to roll over diverse, complicated problems until folks have had time to prioritize the issue personally. The lesson — Invest your emotions wisely!

CHAPTER THIRTEEN

Dollar Scholars — A Closing Word

13
❦

Never think about money the same way! That was our pledge in the beginning. We hope now that you've taken our challenge, you understand why we say you are complete with a personal **Millionaire Code**. You can utilize your strengths and choose to change any thoughts and behavior with money. By using your own financial personality, you're maximizing your pre-wired **Millionaire Code**, not holding yourself back unconsciously or consciously. Remember the warning: Do not ignore personality flaws.

Resolve this year to challenge your weaknesses and create mental breathing room that will unlock your money strengths. So, one more time — here's one last "cheat sheet" for you to use to keep the essence of your financial DNA in mind:

Pleasure Seeking Millionaire Codes:

Ask not how to get something for nothing, but what the investment is worth, long term!

When an investment is worth the price and the risk, instead of rejecting it — "I can't afford it — I already spent it," ponder instead, "How can I afford it?" Reprioritize your spending.

Powerbroker Millionaire Codes:

Ask not *just* how to diversify your money, but how to *focus* investments for greater return!

Instead of trying to control money, focus instead on controlling your relationship with money.

Problem Solving Millionaire Codes:

Ask not *just* how to secure your money, but how to maintain your freedom using money? Instead of avoiding risk, recognize and focus on managing risk.

Peacemaker Millionaire Codes:

Ask not how to *just* play it safe with money, but how to play it smart?

Instead of worrying about what your friends will think of your investment, focus on what's best for you.

The Bottom Line: Each one of the personalities is complete with equal strengths and weaknesses. Allow weaknesses to rule your life, and your life will be fraught with more financial worries and concerns than successes. If, however, you lean toward strengths, you'll find yourself a dollar scholar living the good life with lifetime dues paid and just maybe a secure membership in "The 3.5 Club."

References

Aging and Personality. (September, 2000). *The Harvard Mental Health Letter*, *17*, p. 7.

Alessandra, T., & O'Connor, M. (1996). *The Platinum Rule*. New York: Little, Brown & Co.

Arond, M., & Pauker, S.L. (1999). *The First-Year of Marriage*. New York: Warner Books.

Azar, B. (September, 2002). Searching for genes that explain our personality. *Monitor on Psychology, 33*, pp. 44-46.

Bono, J.E., Boles, T.L., Judge, T.A., & Lauver, K.J. (2002). The role of personality in task and relationship conflict. *Journal of Personality, 70*, pp. 311-344.

Bach, D. (2002). *Smart Couples Finish Rich*. New York: Broadway Books.

Begley, S. (March 27, 2002). The Nature of Nurturing. *Newsweek, 137*, pp. 64-66.

Begley, S. (August 30, 2002). Follow your intuition: The unconscious you may be the wiser half. *Science Journal, Wall Street Journal*, B1.

Begley, S. (September 6, 2002). How do I love thee? Let me count the ways and other bad ideas. *Science Journal, Wall Street Journal*, B1.

Begley, S. (October 11, 2002). Survival of the busiest, parts of the brain that get most use literally expand and rewire on demand. *Science Journal, Wall Street Journal*, B1.

Begley, S. (November 15, 2002). This is your brain. This is your brain on a surging stock. *Science Journal, Wall Street Journal*, B1.

Buckingham, M., & Clifton, D.O. (2001). *Now Discover Your Strengths*. New York: Free Press.

Canli, T., Zhao, A., Desmond, J.E., Kang, E., Gross, J., & Gabrieli, J. (2001). An fMRI study of personality influences on brain reactivity to emotional stimuli. *Behavioral Neuroscience, 115*, pp. 33-42.

Carter, J. (1996). *Living Faith*. New York: Random House

Chambers, O., Reimann, J., & Stanley, C.F. (1992). *My Utmost for His Highest*. Grand Rapids, MI: Discovery House.

Chilton, D. (1998). *The Wealthy Barber*. New York: Prima Publishing.

Clark, J.B., & Burt, E. (March, 2002). Cheap talk does Clark Howard have a deal for you. *Kiplinger's Personal Finance, 56*, pp. 112-115.

Clements, D. (October 16, 2001). Getting going: Rating a broker? Listen to the pickup line. *Wall Street Journal.*

Cole, N., & Diehl, D. (2000). *Angel on My Shoulder: An Autobiography.* New York: Warner Books.

Cooper, J., & Lance, K. (1999). *The Body Code, 4 Genetic Types, 4 Diet Solutions.* New York: Simon & Schuster.

Dunnavant, K. (August, 2001). Talking the Talk: Clark Howard. *Atlanta, 41,* pp. 44-46.

Farrell, W. (1999). *Women Can't Hear What Men Don't Say: Destroying Myths, Creating Love.* New York: JP Tarcher.

Farrell, W. (1993). *The Myth of Male Power: Why Men Are the Disposable Sex.* New York: Simon Schuster.

Farrell, W. (1986). *Why Men Are the Way They Are.* New York: McGraw Hill.

Felton-Collins, V. (1990). *Couples and Money: Why Money Interferes with Love & What To Do About It.* New York: Bantam Books.

Foley, M.E., & Finney, M.I. (2001). *Bodacious: An AOL Insider Cracks the Code to Outrageous Success for Women.* New York: AMACOM.

Fuqua, J.B., & Johnson, T., & O'Briant, D. (2002). *Fuqua: How I Made My Fortune Using Other People's Money.* Atlanta: Longstreet.

Goode, E. (May 19, 2000). Response to stress found that's particularly female. www.nytimes.com/library/national/science/health/051900hth-women-stress.htm.

Heinrichs, J. (December, 2001). People who become words. *Reader's Digest.* p. 132.

Howard, C., & Meltzer, M. (2002). *Get Clark Smart: The Ultimate Guide to Getting Rich from America's Money-Saving Expert.* New York: Hyperion.

Jordan, H. (September 27, 1982). Crisis: The last year of the Carter presidency, part 1. *Newsweek, 100,* pp. 50-61.

Jordan, P. (2000). *The Fitness Instinct: The Revolutionary New Approach to Health Exercise That is Fun, Natural, and No Sweat.* Emmaus, PA: Rodale Press.

Kagan, J. (October, 2000). Adult personality and early experience. *The Harvard Mental Health Letter, 17,* pp. 4-5.

Kennedy, J. (January, 2003). A passion for Plains. *GEMC Georgia, 59,* pp. 15-16.

Kennedy, J. (January, 2003). Jimmy Carter reflects on Plains: A Labor of Love. *GEMC Georgia*, *59*, pp. 17-24.

Kipfer, B. (1992). *Roget's 21ˢᵗ Century Thesaurus*. New York: Dell Publishing.

Kiyosaki, R., & Lechter, S.L. (1998). *Cashflow Quadrant: Rich Dad's Guide to Financial Freedom*. New York: Warner Books.

Kiyosaki R.T., & Lechter, S.L., (2000). *Rich Dad, Poor Dad: What the Rich Teach their Kids about Money – That the Poor and Middle Class Do Not*. New York: Warner Books.

Kiyosaki, R., & Lechter, S.L. (2000). *Rich Dad's Guide to Investing: What the Rich Invest in That the Poor and the Middle Class Do Not*. New York: Warner Books.

Lobb, A. How does your spending stack up? *CNN/Money*, http://money.cnn.com/2002/10/24/pt/millionaire/q_millionaire_expenses/index.htm.

Libet, B. (1985). Unconscious cerebral initiative and the role of conscious will in voluntary action. *The Behavioral and Brain Sciences*, *8*, pp. 529-566.

Littauer, F., & Littauer, M. G (1998). *Getting Along with Almost Anybody: The Complete Personality Book*. Grand Rapids, MI: Baker House Books/Fleming H. Revell Company.

Littauer, F., & Littauer, F. (1997). *After Every Wedding Comes a Marriage*. Eugene, OR: Harvest House Publishers, Inc.

Marcus, A. (July 19, 2002). Anxiety is in the gene. *Healthscout News*. Healthscout.com, #508198.

Matheny, K.B., & McCarthy, C.J. (2000). *Write Your Own Prescription for Stress*. Oakland, CA: New Harbinger Publications.

Olson, D.H., & DeFrain, J.D. (2000). *Marriage and the Family, Strengths and Diversity*. New York: McGraw-Hill.

Paying yourself first, a tool for managing time and risk. (May/June, 2002). *USAA Magazine*, pp. 8-12

Pervin, L.A., & John, O.P. (1999). *Handbook of Personality: Theory and Research* (2ⁿᵈ ed.). New York: Guilford Press.

Pritzker, S., & Greenberg, G. (July/August, 2000). Who wants to be a millionaire? The tragedy of "Sudden Wealth Syndrome." *Psychology Today*, *32*, p. 84.

Robertson, J.C. (1994). *Workaholism* (audio tape). Saginaw, MI: Robertson Institute, Ltd.

Robins, R.W., Fraley, R.C., Roberts, B.W., & Trzesniewski, K.H. (2001). A longitudinal study of personality change in young adulthood. *Journal of Personality*, *69*, pp. 617-640.

Sanders, T. (2002). *Love Is the Killer App: How to Win Business and Influence Friends*. New York: Crown Publishing.

Sapolsky, R. (April 10, 2000). It's not 'all in the genes.' *Newsweek*, *135*, p. 68

Schott, J.W., & Arbeiter, J.S. (1998). *Mind over Money: Match Your Personality to a Winning Financial Strategy*. New York: Little Brown & Company.

Spanos, A. (2002). *Sharing the Wealth: My Story*. Washington, D.C.: Regnery Publishing.

SPECIAL ON HEALTH. (June 28, 1999). *Newsweek*.

Stanley, T.J. 2000. *The Millionaire Mind*. Kansas City: Andrews-McMeel.

Trump, D. (1993). *The Art of the Deal*. New York: Random House.

Thurow, L.C. (1999). *Building Wealth*. New York: HarperCollins.

Weaver, T. (October 4, 2002). Live! From New York's it's. . .Rudy! Blunt ex-mayor tells how to get things done. *Atlanta Journal-Constitution*, p. E1.